Reviews of *T*

'*The Pilo Family Circus* is an excellently coherent act of imagination. It's funny violent and full of bizarre characters ... The plot is full of wonderful grotesqueries and unfolds at a cracking pace ... I was enjoying reading this book so much, I forgot I was meant to review it.' *Sydney Morning Herald*

'The novel, with its elements of fantasy and horror, stands firm as wholly original.' *The Age*

'Peopled with memorable freaks and packed with punchy surprises, it marks Elliott as a writer to watch.' *Good Reading*

This is territory where few Australian novelists have ventured, let alone with Elliott's disquieting composure ... *The Pilo Family Circus* reminds us how far some Australian novelists have left the parochial behind.' *The Bulletin*

'Elliott is to be congratulated for the risks he takes ... *The Pilo Family Circus* displays an adventurousness that is all too rare in contemporary Australian fiction.' *Australian Bookseller & Publisher*

'This is a first novel of real promise. At his best, Elliott writes with a power commensurate with the originality of his vision. It is not just that he has unusually nasty visions to put on the page, but he has the ability to make us share them.' *Times Literary Supplement*

'I couldn't put Elliott's debut novel down. It's fantastic.' *Independent on Sunday*

'This inventive, scary and darkly humorous novel has a dash of Stephen King and a hint of Lovecraft but it is really *sui generis*. It may be a true one-off but that doesn't stop me wanting more.' *The Observer*

ABOUT THE AUTHOR

Will Elliott's first novel, *The Pilo Family Circus* (2006), won five major literary awards, including the coveted Golden Aurealis Award for Best Novel. He was named one of the best young novelists for 2007 by the *Sydney Morning Herald* and was shortlisted for the 2006 International Horror Guild Award for Best Novel. He is currently working on his next book.

STRANGE PLACES

A MEMOIR OF MENTAL ILLNESS

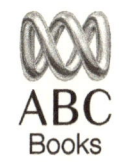

WILL ELLIOTT

ABC Books

The ABC 'Wave' device is a trademark of the Australian Broadcasting Corporation and is used under licence by HarperCollins*Publishers* Australia.

First published in Australia in 2009
by HarperCollins*Publishers* Australia Pty Limited
ABN 36 009 913 517
www.harpercollins.com.au

Copyright © William Elliott 2009

The right of William Elliott to be identified as the author of this work has been asserted by him in accordance with the *Copyright Amendment (Moral Rights) Act 2000*.

This work is copyright. Apart from any use as permitted under the *Copyright Act 1968*, no part may be reproduced, copied, scanned, stored in a retrieval system, recorded, or transmitted, in any form or by any means, without the prior written permission of the publisher.

HarperCollins*Publishers*
25 Ryde Road, Pymble, Sydney, NSW 2073, Australia
31 View Road, Glenfield, Auckland 0627, New Zealand
1–A Hamilton House, Connaught Place, New Delhi – 110 001, India
77–85 Fulham Palace Road, London W6 8JB, United Kingdom
2 Bloor Street East, 20th floor, Toronto, Ontario M4W 1A8, Canada
10 East 53rd Street, New York NY 10022, USA

National Library of Australia Cataloguing-in-Publication data:

Elliott, Will.
  Strange places: a memoir of mental illness/Will Elliott.
  ISBN: 978 0 7333 2352 2 (pbk.)
  Elliott, Will.
  Schizophrenia.
  Schizophrenics – Biography.
  Australian Broadcasting Corporation.
616.898092

Cover photography © Richard Hamilton Smith/CORBIS
Cover design by Natalie Winter
Typeset in 11/18pt ACaslon by Kirby Jones
Printed and bound in Australia by Griffin Press
70gsm Classic used by HarperCollins*Publishers* is a natural, recyclable product made from wood grown in sustainable forests. The manufacturing processes conform to the environmental regulations in the country of origin, Finland.

5 4 3 2   09 10 11 12

AUTHOR'S NOTE

Names have been altered to protect the privacy of people mentioned. Also, I have invented fictional names for medications. Although some medicines were unsuitable for my treatment, they may be the best option for others. It would be irresponsible of me to denigrate or recommend any specific medication.

INTRODUCTION

Where am I?

Sitting at the same scratched blue computer desk, smack bang in the same northern Brisbane suburb everything else happened in. The townhouse is a touch nicer than the shitty little apartment in which my earlier books were produced — that little sweatshop of my own making — but only a touch. Everything has changed, but it sure doesn't look or feel like it. Not sure what I expected … fireworks? Orchestras bursting into song? Tickertape parades? Nope, it's just Tuesday again. Weird.

There are awards on the shelf beside my writing desk. Major ones, not those little certificates that used to arrive in the post and make my day: *Congratulations! You have been shortlisted in such-and-such a short-story competition.* Those were special, in their way, but these awards are different. These say I've butted heads with published authors.

One, two, six of them. Jesus. Three glass plaques, a statuette, two certificates. To look at them makes me feel a little numb. There are copies of my debut novel on the shelf too, the Australian edition and the UK edition, side by side. I've yet to actually read *The Pilo Family Circus* from cover to cover in book format — after all those rewrites, I'm sick of it, frankly. Not everyone feels that way, though. The reviews in the UK were even more glowing than the local reviews. *The Times Literary Supplement*, *Guardian*, *Observer*. It'd do your head in if you were sane to start with.

How did this happen? I mean, *actually* happen? It sounds like the kind of thing you read about happening to someone else. How can something that began as mere thought, dashes and sketches in a notebook, then simply words across a screen, words on printing paper bought from Strathpine's Woolworths for five dollars, on the cheapest possible laser printer bought on a long lay-by, end up for sale in bookshops around the world?

I met up with my Italian translator for coffee a few weeks ago — he wanted to check three specific points of translation that were unclear. I had just got back from a reading tour of Germany. Interviews, readings, photographers, signings, all of it surreal while still as ordinary as a day job. I had answered so many questions that talking about myself became a habit, and it was beginning to bleed into regular conversation ... which is a worry.

I've been on live radio a dozen times, seen my face in all the major newspapers, often with long articles about the book and about me.

My bank account is as unhealthy as ever — what money there is takes a long time to come through in this industry — but I have a literary agent, a publisher, and I'm exchanging mail and phone calls with authors I've long admired as though I'm one of them.

Unless I'm missing some fine print, all these things seem to say 'you've made it'.

But for a while, it didn't look like I *would* make it. When I was twenty-one, for example, being driven to hospital, bug-eyed delusional, convinced my father was an android, that a cataclysmic flood was about to blot out the horizon and annihilate the human race. Or when I was nineteen, freshly dropped out of law school, mind already half unhinged, eagerly sucking down yet another lungful of marijuana smoke to the comfortable sound of water burbling in the bong — unaware that the tendrils of curling smoke worming their way inside me would turn into little whispering demons, chattering away until plain English became meaningless behind their babble. Or when I was in hospital for the second time, driven there after I'd walked out into the backyard to show my parents two wrists red with blood from self-inflicted cuts and an air of 'let's get this over with'. Or in those long, long medicated days in between the frantic highs of psychosis, reassembling a smashed picture of reality sliver by shard — a slow job — wondering the whole time what had hit me, wondering if the world was crazy, or if what they said was true: it was just me. (*All* of it, though? How could *all* of it be delusion and lies?)

At twenty-five, I seemed no closer to making it. Alone in my apartment, rewriting one of my manuscripts yet again, the room hazy with cigarette smoke; filthy coffee cups, paperback books and notepads scattered everywhere; the *click-clack* of fingers going across a keyboard — much faster now than they did back when, in a medicated haze, the idea of writing first occurred. Even by now, moving day by day closer to the moment when a phone call would change everything, the idea of success appeared to move *further* away, not closer — so far it was beyond reach, moving faster than I could run even if my legs weren't cramping up and tired. Hell, maybe the possibility was never there to start with; maybe it was just a delusion prettier than the others had been because it had seemed convincing even when the rest were exposed. Except — just a second, the phone's ringing ...

There was always going to be a catch for making it,

beyond the years of work and the sheer risk taken in spent years. The catch was I'd have to write *this* book, different from the others I'd write, since this one wouldn't be made-up. Somehow, in my bones, I knew when first tapping at a keyboard, writing short stories in the spare room at my parents' house: this was the deal made with fate or God or the devil or Lady Luck or whoever answered those prayers, whoever cleared the roadblocks to allow me to reach this place. *OK then. You'll make it. Now here's the catch ...*

What's this all about, anyway? A memoir? Surely not, at the age of twenty-eight. A self-help book? How to survive schizophrenia, something like that? Gonzo journalism? A shotgun-seat ride down the bumpy roads of mental illness, with yours truly as driver and tour guide, pointing out the landmarks and steering like a qualified lunatic? Buckle up, I guess.

So. The illness. It's taken a back seat at long last, rarely thought of as more than the pills that have to be swallowed nightly. They put you to sleep, make it harder to get up in the morning, make you feel kind of hungover and emotionless for a couple of hours, but that's normal, by now. But the decision to write this means it's in charge again, it seems, for a little while:

Psychosis: Any major, severe form of mental illness, as one in which the sufferer loses connection with external reality leading to personality and behaviour changes.
— Macquarie Dictionary, Fourth Edition.

I had two real, full-blown psychotic episodes, culminating in a diagnosis of schizophrenia at age twenty. By 'episode' I just mean a period of time — weeks or months in this case — spent cut off from reality as previously known. There were other periods which skirted close to psychotic, and in fact probably *were*, except the break wasn't of a kind impossible to cross back from unaided.

The first episode was mistakenly thought to be drug-induced psychosis, something that goes away when drug use ceases. In between the two major episodes were quite a few borderline periods skating between normality and full-blown psychosis, sometimes touching on either extremity in consecutive days. Those were the times when medication seemed like, well, kind of a drag and maybe best put on hold indefinitely. Of course medication *is* a drag, which doesn't help anyone concerned. At times it may seem a worse deal than the whims of the illness.

A psychotic episode moves in stealthily. You cannot see

it coming, even if you've been there before. If you *haven't* been there before, the change is all the more overwhelming — especially, perhaps, because the people around you won't have seen it before either. It can't be overcome by willpower alone, any more than gravity can, which is something I discovered the hard way, like many do. In fact, in the midst of it, you don't even realise you're falling, that anything is out of the ordinary — with yourself, that is. You may have noticed some new enemies, shadowy ones, lurking around every corner, sending oblique signals, dropping hints. You try to seize onto something solid, some reference point, but it's like grabbing at shapes made of smoke. You may suddenly be thrown into some conspiracy which is as real as concrete, though it sounds as wild as some sci-fi TV show. You may hear people speak who aren't actually there, or, as happened in my case, the television or radio may begin sending coded signals, only to you. Likewise song lyrics, newspaper headlines, car licence plates, maybe even shapes in the clouds, are all infused with sinister meanings or grand promises or both.

But you feel normal; you feel fine. You maybe never felt better, never more energetic, more decisive, more switched-on mentally, more important in the scheme of things — unless and until you start to get *scared* by all these things going on around you. Suddenly, you're at centre stage. People speak, but you hear their words differently to everyone else; they are pertaining to that private script in your mind, those conspiracies. You act like a sane person would when the television comes alive and talks to you, *you personally*, referring to your innermost fears: you freak out. It feeds on itself: *they're sending me signals, so they know I'm watching. If they know I'm watching, they can see me right now. They're following me. They're everywhere ...*

And just who is on your side in the midst of all this? Apparently, it's the 'doctor' who wants you to swallow some 'medicine' ... Pull the other one, eh?

When I came out of hospital after the second psychotic episode, I spent some time trying to write this story. That was back in 2001, when I hadn't yet seriously attempted to write a novel, only some short horror stories. My head was not good for much, back then, caught in some weird inertia that happens when a brain once catapulting out of the stratosphere has medicated brakes applied, and slowly sinks back to earth.

The attempt went badly. I got twenty-four thousand words down, but the writing would've failed high school English. Rambling, unstructured, incoherent. Still, it was important — the craziest parts of it were all fresh, had only just happened, and I jotted down a lot of explicit detail which otherwise would've been lost. It has neatly inscribed the whole thing into permanent memory, and it's why no creative licence was required when depicting some of the stranger places I've been.

ONE

There was no indication early on in life that I'd be either a writer or a mental patient, though in retrospect some things point to both, and funnily enough it wasn't until I'd lost it, medically speaking, that any real thought of being a novelist occurred.

As a child, I had a creative side, and though that included writing stories, it expressed itself chiefly in sketches. The stories were perhaps more numerous than would be customary for a child of six or seven, but the main reason I wrote them was so I could illustrate them. Some of these were decent — not a prodigy, but a talent, until harshly worded criticism from an art teacher at school quietly snuffed out any impulse to draw. I was a sensitive lad.

I was also an introvert, in the middle of two brothers, both more outgoing and socially adept. My older brother,

Paul, and I competed fiercely in most things we did. People used to mistake us for twins, until a series of growth spurts saw me shoot skyward. We generally got along, but would often fight like dogs, as though preparing each other for whatever the world outside might throw at us. Our scraps were vicious. I remember knocking his head down on concrete, and remember similar things done to me. I also remember chasing him through the front yard with a huge kitchen knife in my hand — I hadn't ever intended to use it, but he didn't know that. I'd wanted to scare him, and it worked. It wouldn't have been easy then to predict that we would later become close friends.

If you looked into the backyard of our Kallangur home — a regular quarter-acre block dominated by a huge jacaranda tree — you'd see a tall, gangly lad with skin tanned almost ethnically dark, running from a short run-up to bowl a tennis ball at metal stumps set up against the back fence, one after the other, aiming for pace — screw accuracy. A dog named Chockie was invariably in hot pursuit of the ball, already slimy with drool. (Chockie had decided his one purpose in this life was to chase tennis balls, and he did it fanatically, until he was an arthritic limping old man, staggering after the ball at snail's pace.) In winter, I'd use a couple of trees as goal posts and practise kicking a football between them with the same repetitive diligence. By all appearances, a career in data entry was certainly on the cards.

If it was raining, or if wasps had been sighted in the yard — I have a hideously intense phobia of wasps — I'd be in the living room sketching pictures, of people mostly, sometimes inventing comic book characters using Dad's Marvel comics as a guide. Or maybe there'd be a spread of G.I. Joes across the carpet, each a character in some weird sci-fi scenario. Or there might be a little computer chess program balanced across my lap — the damned thing made the same moves every time, and when set on the highest level of difficulty, simply took half an hour to make those same moves. I would most likely be on my own; my brothers Paul and Justin were better friends with each other back then than I was with either.

My father stomped around the house on a Saturday afternoon, sighing in that angry way he had. There was a constant sense of threat in the sound of his footsteps. He was not a friend, did not wish to be liked by us, had a dangerous temper. He was the one who said 'no' when you asked for something, the one who would hit you if you did something bad. If you lied about what you did, he would know and his anger would jump off the scale. So if you lied by reflex, to avoid getting hit, your next lie had better be convincing.

This is not to say his punishments qualified as actual abuse, but I suspect there were occasions when it ranged closer to the borderline than the man intended; this harmed the link between us, making it more tenuous than it might have been. Though an uncommon example, being belted across the backs of my legs with a piece of timber from the barbecue made me genuinely afraid of him from that moment on, made me unable to trust him or relate to him, even when he'd mellowed out in later years.

But, unlike many, he took the job of fatherhood seriously and did his shift for us. To glance at the man's shadow alone would not do him justice; I also know him as a fine human being. There was food on the table because of him, there was a roof over our heads. You need to be told 'no' sometimes, but I didn't realise this at six or seven, and saw only a dangerous creature much bigger than me, feared, best avoided where possible.

There were points of contact. He taught me to play chess when I was four. He made sure the house was filled with encyclopaedias and dictionaries, would help with homework or assignments if we needed it. He instilled in us his own love of music, helped by his enormous record collection. At night, his voice would sometimes take us away to Middle Earth as he read *The Hobbit* or *The Lord of the Rings* to the three of us, doing the voices of the characters superbly. A play made of pure imagination ran across our developing minds, better than a TV show or movie. After each reading I rushed out to Mum, washing up in the kitchen, to give her an avid summary of what had happened in the story that night.

At school, Mrs Grayson would sometimes let me sit apart from the rest of the class to write stories, which were a far higher priority after hearing *The Lord of the Rings*. I began a fantasy epic, complete with drawings, about some dwarfs who wanted to find treasure, but got chased by Nazgul on the way. It's in need of some tweaking, but my agent is going to love it ...

Stories fell off my radar by the age of ten or so, and sport took over, cricket especially. I would watch one-day matches with a calculator in hand, frantically working out required run-rates when the commentators were slow to update them. I spent hours ogling expensive bats in my Greg Chappell Cricket Centre catalogue, hours practising fast bowling in the yard. I'd make Dad laugh with impersonations of famous players, especially English bowler Gladstone Small, who appeared to have no neck at all, or Australian swing bowler Terry Alderman, who seemed to grin like a jackal when he ran in to bowl. I played for a club side and for inter-school teams, and though I didn't exactly set the cricket world on fire, not a childhood memory is sweeter than playing any one of those games.

People say childhood goes fast, but it seems to me those years crawled by, each hour proportionally a bigger slice of your life, as there are fewer to count. I remember afternoons filled to bursting with time, nothing to do, no way to spend it.

I didn't know what to be. Was I an A-grade student? Introverted nerd? Class clown? Jock athlete? Teacher's pet? Rebel? Popular? Outcast? Why not be all of them, try each on like a suit of clothes to see how it fits? Often as not, it depended on the company kept.

Two important things happened in primary school, in terms of the company I keep today. I befriended the chap who would one day be depicted as the main protagonist in my debut novel. Andrew and I got off to a bad start; little chain necklaces were in vogue then, and I broke his the first day we met. Despite that, we made parody lyrics to songs in our music class, and spent many weekend afternoons playing Super Mario Brothers on his Nintendo. At night, we'd sneak out and rock roofs, make prank calls to 'kids help line' or order taxis and pizzas for the houses next door. Andrew and I were the tallest boys in class, and we wound up at the same high school, in the same classes at uni, living in the same share-house and even, at this writing, work in the same office and live in the same suburb, twenty-one years later.

That year, I met a girl named Christine. She had a dental plate and a Smurf watch that she wore up near her elbow as it was too big for her skinny little arm. I'd bump into her again in twenty years or so, after so many life-changing things had already happened. She claims I once belched in her ear in class, which no witnesses have verified. Still, she turned out OK, in the end.

A lot had to happen, though, before she appeared to find me relatively well and living a life vaguely on the right track.

TWO

Dakabin High School was a rougher place then than it is now — the place has changed a lot, by all accounts. In my day tough blue-collar kids went there, not always from good homes. Foul-mouthed girls boasted about losing their virginity well before their fourteenth birthdays. They smoked cigarettes and told tales of abusive stepfathers. Boys would simply beat the shit out of each other; sometimes the girls would do the same. But if a boy made the mistake of hitting a girl, his name would be on the shit-list of the entire school, and he was toast. A roaming pack would chase him down in the lunch hour. A couple of years before I started, there was an incident where a kid was thrown unconscious on to the train tracks after a fight and left to die. I did not thrive in such an environment.

Stealing from shops became my favoured hobby. This was nothing new. The first incident I remember happened when my brothers and I were quite young, after a trip to the beach, when Mum took us to a little corner store to get an ice-cream. Some goodies were pocketed experimentally, and we got away with it. From then on, we'd swipe the odd Mars Bar or pack of gum occasionally — nothing major, just a little bonus when opportunity presented itself.

By high school, though, me and my friends were doing a circuit of the small shops along Kallangur's Anzac Avenue and going home with our school bags full of loot, from blocks of chocolate to bottles of ice-cream topping, from dirty magazines to stuff we didn't even especially *want*. It was incredibly easy to steal. I walk into a shop now and wonder how the hell we did it, in broad daylight, in a shop full of customers, walking right past the crowded newsagency checkout with magazine-shaped bulges down the front of our shirts. How? Maybe the blatancy of it *was* the camouflage.

I sold the porno mags at school for a couple of dollars each, even took orders every now and then. For a while, it was a tidy little business venture. We soon got cocky and brazen. In one shop, I filled my backpack with KitKats, scooping them in by the handful. Andrew and I rode out to a park to tally them — more than thirty-five in one hit. Far more than we could eat. We stuffed ourselves, threw a whole lot of them in the South Pine River (fearful of being caught with the evidence), then went back for more, just to see if we could top our score. This time a company rep saw me piling them from the display bin into my bag while Andrew watched nervously. The rep looked at us, wide-eyed with shock, then turned away and left us to it. I kept scooping the KitKats, then we ran. We rode our bikes back to the park and counted them: over seventy. Most went into the river.

We spent a lot of time at the local shops playing a coin-operated game, 'Double Dragon'. Back then Kallangur was home to bevans, tough teenagers who wore flannelette shirts, listened to Guns N' Roses and hung around the shops at night, drinking cask wine (or 'goon') in car parks, sometimes fighting or destroying a fence. By day, they smoked and bummed around the shops. I'd steal packets of biscuits for them. We'd go out onto the footpath beside the very shop we'd stolen from, eat them, then go back in and play some more Double Dragon until we got hungry again.

Of course this fun had to end. The Kallangur Foodstore must have noticed its missing KitKats, for that was the shop I got busted in a few weeks later. There'd been a narrow escape just the day before from a shop in Petrie which was another favoured haunt of ours. I'd only just made it to my bike in time, having had to yank my shirt out of the checkout lady's fist. It was a pretty clear signal — fun's over — but I didn't listen.

The next day, still somewhat shaken, I decided to settle my nerves by taking one of the easiest items to steal, a block of chocolate. No sweat, into the school bag. Out the door I went, straight to my bike in the rack.

'Excuse me. Excuse me …' A burly female checkout attendant invited me to come back into the shop as I got on my bike. She came straight for me, almost within arm's reach and I was too taken aback to bolt for it. I played innocent, followed her back inside, where she opened my bag. I tried to run but she grabbed me and wouldn't let go. She took me to a back room and sat by the door, her face sympathetic as we waited for the cops to come.

When Mum saw me in the back of the police car, it sounded at first like she'd burst out laughing … but no, not quite. You'd think she'd just been told I was dead.

I don't know where this wildness came from. I was lashing out at something, or someone. It wasn't just stealing. From about twelve to fourteen, I moved on from relatively innocent antics like prank calls and rocking roofs to starting fires, slashing car tyres, even breaking into a school demountable building by sliding out enough glass slats from the louvre windows to climb through. I think Dakabin had set me on a downward spiral; it's hard to tell in retrospect where it would've stopped.

It was in year nine that the Tucker kids, who lived on our street, began following me home from school. For some time we'd been engaged in a minor neighbourhood feud, beginning with a fight during a football game at the local park. Insults would be traded as we rode our bikes past their house on our way to the shops. My brothers and I would leave a dead toad in their letter box; they'd leave a fish on our doorstep. When reinforcements arrived in the form of our cousin Mark, visiting from Clermont, we saved up a day's worth of piss in an old milk bottle and poured it into their cat's bowl, which they left below their front steps. All in good fun, as long as you don't ask my mother, who developed an ulcer during this time, worrying about what could go wrong.

The Tucker boys went to the same high school as us, and it was then that things become a little more serious. They fell in with one of the rough crowds, which Dakabin had in abundance. My brothers and I had friends, but no one who would stand up to those guys. The fifteen-minute walk was a long one when there were four or five bloodthirsty enemies following. 'Hit me. Hit me. C'mon, arsehole, hit me.'

I'd slink around school, feeling hunted, avoiding places I knew they might be, always checking over my shoulder for danger. This wasn't the only flavour tasted in the early years of high school, but it was easily the strongest.

In the classroom, maths was my thing, at the expense of every other subject. For some reason, I only studied hard for maths, content to merely scrape by in everything else. My English teacher said she saw a potential B-plus student languishing away.

That changed. About the time my mother got fed up with Dakabin and began initiating a switch of schools, Dad told me about a book he was reading, set in a giant castle. Some subjects — music, books, chess — tapped into a well of enthusiasm in him that gushed over the space between us, and we'd momentarily seem to be on a different level, before settling back into our habitual uneasy distance. 'The castle itself is like a character in this book,' he said. 'And the characters have strange names, like Prunesquallor and Sepulchrave.'

For a fourteen-year-old, as yet no great chops in English, the Gormenghast trilogy by Mervyn Peake was heavy going, a big step up from Dean Koontz novels or Roald Dahl. I stayed up late with a bedside light on, dictionary at hand, doing battle with new long words on every page. The opening volume, *Titus Groan*, was determined to shake me off. *You don't belong in these pages*, it taunted. *Come back in a few years.*

I read late into the night, even on school nights. *Titus Groan* threw multiple four- and five-syllable words into its sentences — *long* sentences, poetic sentences, each so laden with meaning, imagery and artistry it felt like my brain had to physically stretch to hold those sentences in, straining to patiently massage everything out of them, determined not to miss a thing Mervyn Peake had meant. Actually having to *work* to get to that author's story, not having it spoon-fed, was a new experience, and I was unprepared for how rewarding it could be, if the payoff was powerful. I was absolutely lost in that huge crumbling castle, the bizarre rituals of the place, watching Steerpike's evil plans unfold, watching Flay's war with the chef, Swelter, the tragic unfolding madness of the Earl, Sepulchrave. Words — words can do *this*? My head was filled with words, so full they spilled out of me.

I finished the trilogy and began rereading my favourite parts. My mind was digesting the most incredible, massive feast it had ever beheld. Little machines and gears were being switched — I could feel it, again it was almost a physical sensation. The trilogy became ... not quite an obsession, but not far from it.

Suddenly school assignments were child's play. Words were pouring out. In second gear I could pull an A-minus on an essay, twenty minutes tops, barely even paying attention to what I wrote. This kid named Worthington paid me twenty bucks to do an assignment for him — my first paid gig, serious cheese at fifteen. I got him a B-plus on purpose, as he'd been failing the subject. He demanded his money back, having expected an A. My first critic.

A career in writing? The thought entered my head here and there throughout high school. I even wrote a half-decent Lovecraftian horror story for the school magazine. The impulse to write that story had just come to me from nowhere, after reading some Lovecraft at seventeen, also borrowed from my dad's bookshelf. But the idea of being a writer never took hold long enough for serious examination. I'm a tad slow on the uptake, sometimes.

Thanks to Mervyn, every subject that required writing could now be passed with minimal effort. It was kind of cheating; if you knew words, you could make it sound like you knew a subject even if you didn't, just by feel and some very general phrases with pretty wording. Naturally, my maths grades plummeted. I never got higher than a C thenceforth.

* * *

On moving to Pine Rivers High School at fifteen, I settled down a bit, but I don't mean to suggest I was the model pupil. I would hurl chairs or aluminium bins over the edge of a verandah into the garden below, for the amusement of the class waiting down there for their teacher. The class loved it, but it was grounds for instant suspension had any authority figure seen it.

I was suspended once for fighting, to match a suspension already received at Dakabin for the same offence. There were various games played in class which I'm sure caused some teachers to loathe me. In one, we would ask deliberately stupid questions, often utterly irrelevant to the lesson being taught. The winner, the dumbest question that I recall was asked during an economics lesson, was: 'Sir? Are sharks hungry?' Another game was called 'Buh'. In this, one person cleared his throat. The next cleared his a little louder. You passed around the room making some little cough or remark or exclamation, a touch louder each time. The winner was the last one who dared. I usually won the game, but spent a fair amount of time sitting outside the room in disgrace as a result.

In year eleven, a gang I'd somehow offended began giving me the Dakabin treatment. Pine Rivers wasn't as rough a school as Dakabin, but it did have a reputation for lads ganging up on each other — while Dakabin had 'bevans', Pine Rivers had 'homies', who listened to gangsta rap and emulated their idols as best they could by forming aggressive little cliques.

The gang would wait for me at the train station, once decking me on the way there after cricket practice, once pulling a butterfly knife. My dad called the ringleader's dad and asked him to please cut the shit or police would be brought in. They cut the shit, but the sight of a knife meant I'd had enough. Looking over your shoulder for threats gets really, really tiresome.

I shaved my head and began hanging around a group of skinheads, a couple of whom were students. We went out one night and sprayed some swastikas at a local park. Another night, they stomped some guy judged to be a 'homie' gang member by his style of dress. I'm happy to say I wasn't involved in the violence; that happened quickly, as I ran down the street to catch up with the rest of them who were in hot pursuit of their victim. It was all over in a few seconds. I don't know what I would have done if I'd been closer — maybe joined in.

After they'd kicked him around a bit, we turned to leave. To the group's astonishment, the victim stood up and called us pussies for taking him four to one. He dared us to meet him in town some time with a few of his crew, see how tough we were then.

The guy leading us around, Bryce, was a couple of years older than the rest of us, charismatic but hard as nails. He was baffled. The beating had been relatively light until the guy got back up; just a bit of a touch-up. Bryce pulled out a miniature baseball bat he kept up his jacket sleeve, called the guy a fucking idiot, then quickly smacked him twice in the head with it: *thock, thock*. This time he stayed down.

Word spread. I was left alone, which was a nice feeling.

The skinheads knew a few of the army guys I'd begun to hang around — 'army guys' because that's where most of them ended up. A lot of them had dads who were Vietnam vets. Though sternly disciplined at home, they were often quite wild — two of my friends once took a rifle to school at night and shot up a demountable building for kicks. We chuckled to ourselves as the local newspaper reported 'gang activity'. For months afterwards we picked little smashed bullets out of holes in the classroom walls. 'Found another one, Miss!'

One morning at the train station, one of the army guys happened to see me kissing a Chinese girl I'd known at Dakabin. I must've forgotten the part about mixing races; at sixteen or seventeen, a girl's pretty much a girl, especially when you haven't kissed that many. He reported my crime to Bryce, who apparently was astonished to hear of it. The skinheads didn't come after me — I never saw Bryce again — but I wasn't invited out to go stomping anymore.

The army guys were good mates, for the most part. Which is not to say good influences.

As year twelve drew to an end we discovered inebriation and found it a noble pursuit. There was a grassy little hill out the back of Westfields that had once been a BMX track. On weekends we'd gather there and swig bourbon from the bottle like it was lemonade, daring each other to take longer pulls, not quite understanding the nature of bourbon, but on a hard learning curve.

'Cones' were next on our to-do list. Sometimes we'd sneak down to the creek behind the school's far oval. Hidden in the undergrowth were a couple of Coke-can bongs; simply aluminium cans with little holes punched into them. You laid the drug across the holes, lit it up and sucked the smoke through the can's mouthpiece. I'd been down there a couple of times to watch, fascinated, as the weed smokers went through the ritual of chopping the goods up in a little clay bowl with scissors, mixing with a pinch of tobacco, packing and smoking.

When I finally joined in, I sucked at the harsh hot smoke but nothing happened. I pretended to be stoned.

The next time, same deal. *What's the attraction here?* I wondered.

The third time did it. I took a very long pull and held it. Suddenly my brain slipped inside a bubble. My laugh came from far away. I tried to speak but could not. It felt strange to be inhabiting a body at all, like I'd momentarily lost control of a giddy puppet made of flesh, absolutely lost contact — I could hear, distantly, the voices of my friends but not understand a word. My head was trying to float away from my body. Some barrier had been broken down at last; here it was. The drug and I had shaken hands and been properly introduced.

It took a long time to come back within reach of sobriety, enough to sneak back into school. The experience didn't scare me, not in the way I needed to be scared, but the clouded, hungover feeling that came the next day didn't make me rush to try it again, not with exams coming up. Alcohol was easier to get hold of anyway, so pot wasn't a common occurrence, not yet. It had been something, though, that feeling. I intended to go there again.

I'd also just had the marvellous idea of taking up cigarette smoking, having tried my first out of sheer bewilderment as I watched some girls in my class smoke while waiting for a train. It was such a stupid idea, I had to see why people did it. I tried it and — whoa — my head spun pleasantly for about twenty minutes. Peace pipe, all right. The habit was enforced after the odd bong session, because a cigarette after a cone gives the cone a nice little kick. The smokes have a nice little kick on their own, too, which remains the case for, say, the first couple of hundred you smoke. They go by pretty quickly.

School's end was an exciting time. My marks were merely decent, not as good as they could have been, thanks to my new pastimes. The big wide world approached. Uni and beyond. Driving cars, casual jobs, eighteenth birthdays, nights on the town, hormones at the wheel. Alcohol was excellent and novel and exciting — three-dollar bottles of Passion Pop got the job done. Schoolies Week was a blur of emotion, happiness, running into old friends from Dakabin on the beach, old friends from primary school, faces you never thought you'd see again, faces I've never seen since. Drunk, drugged or otherwise, we were bright young sparks of life, swarming across the beach at midnight, living days and nights you wished you could freeze still and keep somewhere safe, to step back into every now and then.

But when they're gone, they're gone.

THREE

I'd never dreamed of being a lawyer, just kind of drifted into law school since it was just within reach of my high school results. The army guys mostly went south to ADFA, the military academy in Canberra.

My justice studies double degree meant a heavy workload, and a steep climb out of high school into academia. Justice studies subjects were easily enough passed. The lecturers weren't shy about their political opinions, so it wasn't hard to give them what they wanted. Law, however, was all content, research, readings, finding obscure passages in a library full of tomes. I'd get out of bed at 5 am to make a long trek into the city for law classes, then off to the other campus for an afternoon justice studies lecture, then back again for a night time law tutorial. The workload was manageable if you stayed ahead of it; slip behind a little in readings, on an assignment, or miss a tute, and suddenly you were swamped, barely keeping abreast. But even while delivering pizzas on the side, I passed my subjects, though sometimes narrowly.

Marijuana wasn't on the menu just then; that was something we'd messed around with during the holidays before uni started; blasting our heads with booze and pot, going on impromptu camping trips that became giggling smoke fests, all of us stoned, talking shit, carving tribal weapons out of fallen tree branches. The highs were never as intense or otherworldly as that first big one by the creek at school, but there was plenty of laughing to movies or zonking out over PlayStation games, plenty of munchie runs to the servo to load up on Pringles.

The clouded feeling the day after a smoke was the reason I avoided the drug at uni. It was a feeling of slightly unnatural haziness, like fog layered thick across my mind. But after first year was done and dusted, the long summer break presented a chance to cut loose. There was no shortage of co-conspirators; wherever you went, someone had pot or wanted it. You'd eagerly hop in a car with people you'd just met, often slimy types, everyone bound by the same mission. It is the first rung down on a ladder to seedy subterranean places, but ground level's still close enough that you don't have to worry.

I'd discovered nightclubbing, too, and the pursuit of female flesh, more often than not a fruitless hunt, since older guys were more desirable. Brain-hammering drinking sessions were also the norm. Mid-week? Why not? You'd choose between the two drugs for the night: alcohol was as easy to get as a trip to the bottle-o, but its effects more boring and predictable than pot. Decisions, decisions.

When uni rolled around again, after a few months of rock-star-like inebriation, I was just not up for it anymore. I was surrounded by committed, ambitious, hard-working students, all eager to get somewhere and do the required work. I wasn't one of them. I had no inclination to cease smoking pot this time around, either, despite its effect on study. I began asking myself: *What am I doing here? I don't belong. I never wanted to be a fucking lawyer.*

I dropped some subjects to begin with, then the whole course. I got a casual job at a service station, in addition to delivering pizza. Meanwhile, the couch, marijuana, computer games and much trouble awaited.

There were no outward signs of trouble on the horizon that I could see, but, insidiously, marijuana moved in to stay. I did not attribute my dropping out of uni to the influence of pot, though it certainly played no small part.

Motivational speakers do not advise you to pass the duchy, I am guessing.

My brother Paul — who wanted to be an actor — worked in a bank, and through his contacts there could score cheap weed for the rest of us. Paul, bless him, was never able to keep track of who owed him for last week's hooter; the drug plays havoc with short-term memory.

We'd smoke at home for the most part, or, if the parents were around, go for a drive to a nearby lookout tower where, at the top of an iron ladder, there was a wooden platform with room for five or six. It was a dangerous climb down stoned, but when you were up there, the view of the suburb spread out below was amazing, a sea of lit windows and streetlights. You could pretend to be in another world and believe it.

There were no warning bells to indicate the drug was bad for us. It was fairly benign, this low-concentrated 'bush weed', not like the hydroponic stuff crossbred for dramatic concentration of THC, pot's active ingredient. We'd smoke the hydro when we could be bothered getting it, but it was more expensive, meant cross-town wild-goose chases, and your stash wouldn't last long. This stuff was cheap and you got a huge bagful. The high was a relaxing little buzz. We would play around on guitars, pen lyrics to songs, and talk of forming a band.

Pot enhanced other things; songs sounded better, food tasted better, simple conversations seemed deep and profound. People's words contained many meanings, so many you lost track of the most obvious; what quaint mystery. Then you came down, slept it off, hazy hangover and all, and things were normal again, for the moment.

There was not yet the sense of distant foreboding, while high — that sense of very real danger encroaching on what was safe and fun. That sinister force, whatever it was, was still distant, not yet close enough for me to hear its footsteps or see its shadow up ahead, though moving closer with each inhale.

Daytime was for TV and computer games, each day a pleasant, predictable non-event. I would hang around the local Dominos, where my friend Brad, from Dakabin, worked. I worked for a different pizza joint a few suburbs away. We'd discuss ways to rip them off as Brad cooked up a pizza for me on the house. He opted for the 'direct theft' method: place a fifty from the till in your back pocket when no one was looking. He got away with doing this every shift for an inexplicably long time. My scheme was a little more elaborate and gradual, and involved pretending to offer discounts to customers. If a pizza was late, you could offer them five bucks off or, in extreme cases, a free pizza. I'd mark discounts for several customers on the receipt but charge full price, keeping the difference. On a busy night, like State of Origin night or New Year's, you could scoop off seventy dollars easy.

Andrew and I weren't seeing much of each other around this time. I'd helped organise a major party at Andrew's place while his parents were away, and the house was trashed pretty badly. The trampoline was destroyed, the wine collection raided, there were burn marks around the wooden pool deck from soda-bomb explosions, and someone had practised his golf swing in the yard with empty stubbies, rather than a golf ball. The next phone bill showed calls to European countries and sex lines. Andrew was justifiably pissed. So Brad was now my main smoke-buddy, one of a cast of about a dozen.

By night, Brad would come hang around at the service station where I worked, waiting for my shift to end. As trade for the free pizzas, I turned a blind eye to the odd pack of smokes that ended up in his pocket without payment.

It was good to have company at the servo — the place had been robbed a couple of weeks prior to my starting there. We were on a street corner in the quiet suburb of Narangba, a place then half bush, half suburbia. Anyone who's worked at a servo at night knows the unique kind of lonely tension you feel, how glad you are to see customers, the nervousness after they leave, the sweet relief when your shift ends uneventfully. The woman who worked the shift before mine had jumped and nearly screamed the first time I walked in; someone had stuck a gun in her face for the hundred dollars or so in the till, and she was now a jittery wreck. There were no cameras in the shop — our security was a claw-hammer under the counter. Welcome to your new job.

I was told to make sure it looked like I was working at all times. The shop's owner, a gruff man in his seventies, reputedly had informers who would slowly drive past at night to make sure you were busy. The way the servo women spoke when giving these dire warnings, their eyes wide with fright, their awed whispers, indicated that to be seen slacking off was a terrible crime indeed. *Christ*, I thought, *it's a servo. What's the big deal? Does he whip you, or what?*

On the positive side, no one had told me not to steal. Cigarettes, magazines, drinks, anything from the hot-food kitchen I presided over. After the initial cleaning was done, I'd sit in the corner of the shop, out of view of the rumoured spies and informers, smoking, with an iced coffee in hand and a *Playboy* across my lap, watching time tick away. No security cameras had its advantages.

STRANGE PLACES

After work, Brad and I would hit a bong somewhere. For supposedly casual fun, our behaviour was a little desperate when it came time to score — and it was always time to score. At first, pot and alcohol had been level-pegging; now, we needed smoke almost daily. There were many ludicrous late-night dashes across town. The dealer at Strathpine's out of stock, but he knows someone on the south side who can fix you up. That dealer's not home, but someone knows this guy out at Caboolture. The Caboolture guy doesn't deal anymore, but he knows someone else in Strathpine. That Strathpine dealer only sells quarter-ounces, but he knows someone …

Three hours later it's back home to chop up, conversation revolving almost entirely around weed, its quality, how it compared to last time's, remember that skunk at the party a while back? Then the bong does its first round and other things are discussed, like the band we're going to form, possible band names, who's going to play what. Paul hitting us up for money we owed from last week's supply, us denying all knowledge. The backdrop, a thick fog of pungent exhaled smoke, muffled barking coughs, and the stereo inside playing Faith No More or Primus quietly, a PlayStation running Tekken 3.

* * *

As the weeks passed, all other activities occurred with a weed session. A party wasn't a party without it — you didn't need a party if you had it.

My nineteenth birthday party was saturated in marijuana. Paul's friend Doug, another aspiring actor, brought an ounce by himself. Justin, Brad and Paul's work mates all had a stockpile for the occasion; it would have rivalled Woodstock. I was shouted joints all night. There was an endless procession of people sneaking up the back, out of view of my parents, to get high. The backyard hose was decimated. The drinkers were outnumbered by red-eyes.

Next day, paraphernalia littered the back yard. Dad asked angrily who it belonged to. We blamed it on Brad's little brother, who was then banned from our house. It didn't bother us; he rarely bought his own.

All kinds of people gravitate towards the drug. You become part of a network — by necessity — if you intend to smoke it a lot, unless you've got a green thumb. A friend of Brad's appeared in our midst, Craig, who the rest of us privately nicknamed Gutterboy. There was something faintly rat-like about the guy's face, his speech and manner alternating between shifty and obsequious, too quick to laugh at your jokes, too obvious in his attempts to ingratiate, then ask for favours. I never liked the guy, never trusted him, but on those nights when Paul couldn't fix us up with some gear, Gutterboy knew of many, many dealers.

Brad and Gutterboy weren't of a philosophical bent when stoned; they talked about weed, dealers, cops, fights. That conversation made me uneasy, made what we were doing seem dark and dangerous. Whenever talk steered that way I would be constantly checking the road for police cars, certain one would pull up at any second.

Gutterboy had no love for Paul's mild bush weed — it had to be top shelf, and soon we shared this opinion. Our tastes were beginning to run to something stronger, like hydro or skunk weed (so named for its powerful smell, indicating high THC content). You gauged its quality by the strength of its odour; if you could smell it while it was still in your pocket, you were about to become thoroughly wrecked. Mindful of this, some dealers were not above spraying insect killer on their product so it smelled like quality stuff. Sometimes there'd be a trace of speed in there, too; that gave it a kick. We sat up on the tower's platform, overlooking the suburb below, and passed the bong around, night after night.

The effect the stronger weed was having on me didn't really seem pleasant as time passed. After the brief high

— a head-spinning buzz — thoughts plunged to obscurity. It made me tired and hazy, like I'd inhaled exhaust fumes. Though ceasing use never occurred to me, not for one second, after we smoked, I always just wanted to go home where it was safe.

Our routine was now established. Every night around six, my brother Justin and I would expect a call from Brad. He'd come over, Gutterboy in tow. We'd feed some half-baked innocent-sounding cover story to parents — off to read the Bible at Brad's place, Ma — then arrange to score. We all came to know each other's paydays. It was amazing how, no matter how broke everyone was, we would still wind up with something to smoke. A few times we were reduced to scraping the sticky black residue from the hose of a used bong. It did the job, after a fashion, but not very well.

My paranoia while stoned was now almost a fixture — the guys came to expect it, and joke about it. But things progressed further. At work, I found myself worrying more and more about armed robbery. The servo was so lonely and quiet at night, so vulnerable. Several times, suspicious-looking customers had me close to panic. It was an immense relief when Brad and Gutterboy arrived towards the end of each shift.

STRANGE PLACES

The things I'd stolen, drinks and such, began to play on my mind too. I began to wonder if there really were security cameras after all. I'd inspect the ceiling, peering at each mark on the roof ... Could that be a camera? They can be microscopic in size now, after all ...

It had begun.

FOUR

Our rock band morphed from a stoned idea into a reality. One of my younger brother's friends, Tony, became another regular in our bong sessions. He was a fairly agreeable type, didn't say a whole lot, liked the same music we liked, respected stoner etiquette (shout and be shouted) and played the guitar. Another of Justin's friends played drums. Justin himself played bass. The three of them at some point coalesced and officially became *a band*. My older brother Paul volunteered for vocalist duties. This didn't leave anywhere for me to slot in, something I was acutely aware of from the get-go.

Tony would bring his guitar over to our place. We'd smoke up, then mess around on the instrument. When we were bent, it all sounded fantastic. Tony made some quite decent riffs, nice chunky heavy sounds. Paul started writing song lyrics, Justin and Tony started playing around together, making the beginnings of songs. I went to these early rehearsals, wishing I'd learned to play an instrument when I was younger so I could be a part of it. About the only thing I could do in a band was sing — not that I'd never sung before, but the idea of singing and, particularly, writing lyrics seemed, suddenly, like a calling, like *destiny*. Before marijuana, this had never occurred to me for a moment.

I remember giving an impassioned speech to Justin, telling him that we could really make it big, if we wanted to. We just had to make that one decision that yes, we were going to go for this like our lives depended on it. I sounded like a street-corner preacher. I pointed to the Metallica and Chili Peppers posters on his bedroom wall and said that every one of those guys had made such a decision; if we did the same, then *we* would be up on that wall. Embarrassed, Justin muttered, 'All right already, I get it — just shut up about it, would you?'

From then on our pot sessions had a theme: the band. If Paul was late for a rehearsal, I wouldn't hesitate to pick up the microphone and stand in for him. I couldn't sing, but the beauty of metal is you don't have to. Screams will do it, and I could certainly scream. Of course every jam session began with passing around the bong. Stoned lyrics were the best kind.

Though I badly wanted to join this band, wanted to replace my older brother in it, things between Paul and I only started getting tense when I had a look at his song lyrics, which he'd leave lying around the place in an exercise book. I knew what they meant. The words were directed at me. I *just knew*; there were a lot of things, lately, that I *just knew*. Many of his songs centred on gloating that he was the singer of the band, while I was sitting on the sideline watching. I could see the future mapped out: these guys would be huge, and I'd be a mere roadie, hauling their amps around while they lived the high life. He was going to sing these words in front of everyone, all this coded stuff about me. It may have been in code, but it was still pretty obvious, and I was sure everyone else perceived the insults, too. It made me seethe with anger.

On the drive home from work one day, a car sat at the end of our street. It was just … sitting there. I slowed down to get a look at the driver, and was petrified when I realised it was a cop. His car was a bombed-out and dented white sedan, and he wasn't in uniform, just a light blue business shirt, but I *just knew* it was a cop. He was monitoring our comings and goings, keeping track of our drug dealings.

Back at the house, Justin and Tony were smoking hooter out the back. I joined them. After I'd had my hit, head clouded and spinning, I looked around at the trees past the field next to our backyard. Our house seemed so out in the open, so exposed. I could sense people in the trees, snapping surveillance shots of us.

'You ever think they're watching us?' I asked the guys.

'Who?'

'Cops.'

A knowing, amused look passed between them.

I was getting worried but they didn't seem to care. 'Come on, man, put the bong away,' I said. I snatched it off the table and hid it in the garden. Out there in the trees ... *anyone* could be out there, watching. They didn't understand the risk we were taking. I ushered them inside and closed the blinds. Then I went into my room, and thought about Paul. I started writing lyrics of my own, angry lyrics about him, returning serve. They weren't just words, of course — they seemed to me more like spells.

I warned the guys not to talk about drugs over the phone. I felt pretty sure our line was tapped. Little noises I heard during calls might have given it away. When I called Brad I would try to talk in code, never saying anything directly drug-related. He found it kind of funny and played along.

This notion I had that 'they' were 'on to us' grew when Brad was caught smoking pot by the lake in

Petrie. He'd pulled in for a cone in the car park on his way home from Dominos one afternoon. The police found him with a bong and a small amount of weed. This proved I'd been right to worry. From then on I enforced the secrecy rules with an iron fist. When I heard Paul arrange a deal on the phone in plain English, I furiously chastised him. Paul was surprised; where had this hostility come from? Everything about him was starting to aggravate me, his lyrics most of all. When the guys got together he'd bring his book of songs. I'd have a read. They were so *blatantly* directed at me, it was getting more and more obvious. I answered in kind in my own notebook. It seemed a very important battle. My greatest fear was that these guys would crack it big at any moment, without me on board. They'd barely written a full song yet, they only rehearsed maybe once a week, but there was no doubt in my mind this nightmare scenario would play out.

'Why are you so upset?' someone might have asked. 'What makes you so sure he's writing about you?'

I just knew.

Meanwhile, at the service station, each shift brought a new level of anxiety. The feeling was growing that I was being watched there — by passing cars, by people in the

STRANGE PLACES

houses across the road, by cameras hidden in the ceiling. My boss and his spies were everywhere. And I was more and more convinced that there was going to be a robbery. One night a suspicious-looking van pulled in, and two crim-looking types came in to buy chewing gum. I was certain they were scoping the place for a robbery. They'd checked out the ceiling for cameras, looked in the till when it opened. I jotted down their number-plate as they drove off and called the police.

Ironically enough, the police got in touch next day and said that van *had* been recently used in a robbery on the south side.

I could stand it no more. I quit the servo job and applied for a position as a night filler for Woolworths. I went along for the interview supremely confident. Just lately I'd been on top of the world. I was saying the right thing at the right time wherever I went. It was like some higher sense was guiding me through everything while I stood back and watched. I have since heard this is not uncommon before the onset of a psychotic episode.

I was in better physical shape than ever before, built like an athlete. I had almost no body fat, my shoulders and arms were toned from push-ups and curls. I made a great impression on the woman interviewing me.

'What made you want to leave study?' she asked.

'Well, to me it seems that university is designed to teach people to think, and I already know how to think.' It was the perfect answer, delivered without hesitation. Stuff like that was just bursting out of my mouth everywhere I went.

Although my job was as a night filler, my first couple of shifts were during the day. A manager named Adam showed me around the store, and assured me that there was room in the company to climb the ladder. 'Woolworths is going places,' he said.

'Yeah, I noticed,' I said, as in, W*hy else would a mover and shaker like me be here?* But it wasn't just an act; I believed myself, too. Everything I said seemed to be the right thing to say … but what *was* this higher power speaking for me? My every action, every word, felt like a purposeful statement, as though carefully considered. But it was all spontaneous. I began to think that I knew exactly what I was doing *after* the fact; even if I did say something dumb, it would seem to me that it had been deliberate, to make some point, a tactical masterstroke.

Walking out of the shopping centre after my first day on the job I ran into someone from high school — Lisa. I didn't recognise her at first with her beaming confident smile; in school she'd been overweight and shy. She'd once dared me to wear make-up in a lunch break and I'd done it, walking past the tough kids waving at them. She'd lost a lot of weight and didn't look bad at all, although somehow the weight loss had actually harmed her previous relationship, causing it to end. She was on the market again. She worked at the newsagency in the same shopping complex.

After some small talk, she invited me back to her place; she was living in a caravan park two minutes away. She did most of the talking. I was cautious, unsure of why she should suddenly appear in my life like this. Still, I spent the night and woke up with a girlfriend. From her point of view, her timing was … interesting.

Things began to change pretty quickly.
What the hell is this? I wondered.

I'd just arrived home from my second shift at Woolworths. I stared at the television, not quite believing what I'd just seen. Justin and Tony were on the couch beside me, both stoned, but I hadn't smoked anything yet, which was what made this especially strange — not that anything like this had happened before, even when stoned. I looked over at the guys to see if they'd noticed, but they showed no reaction. Why? It had been so obvious. Were they in on it too? The way they sat there laughing along at some private joke made me wonder.

It came from a commercial for some TV soap or other. The voiceover was describing the plot of tonight's episode — only it wasn't. It was describing the day I'd just had. There were references to a conversation I'd had with Adam at work, about the marketing of Coca-Cola in the drinks aisle. 'Always' was the Coke slogan in those days, and we'd been discussing the placement of fridge magnets which had the word *Always* on them, to subliminally encourage people to buy Coke. I'd spotted the marketing tactic and mentioned it to Adam. He'd reacted strangely, I thought at the time, as if I wasn't supposed to have noticed the fridge magnets, much less commented on them.

The TV show's plot description ran something like:

Will Darren and Sofia's relationship survive the long distance?

He's sacrificed it all for his dream job. This could be the chance he's been waiting for...

This line struck me:

... but you can't ALWAYS get what you want.

I sat wide-eyed. The words, the way they were phrased, the way they were *emphasised* ... it was talking to *me*, directly, about what I'd said at work a few hours ago. It was a threat, a warning — my conversation with Adam at work had displeased 'them', whoever they were.

The logic ran like this: *They sent me a signal. They must therefore know I am watching television right now. How do they know this? They must be able to see me. How? There must be a camera in the television.*

Further: *How did they know about my conversation at work, or anything else? Did work tell them, or were they following me around? Are they watching me everywhere I go?*

They. Who, though? The company ... Which one? Woolworths? Coca-Cola? Both of them together? The government? The police? The TV network? Who?

Tony and Justin were talking about a party somewhere, with maddening casualness, as though nothing had happened. *Play along*, they almost seemed to be saying. So I tried to put it out of my mind.

Tony suggested we head outside for another cone or two. It sounded like a good idea. With the smoke in my system the picture blurred. We went to a party in someone's backyard. I kept to myself while the guys went to a park across the road to smoke pot. In the backyard were groups of people I'd never seen before. I somehow knew they worked for Woolworths, and that they were very displeased with me. From their body language I discerned threats.

Were they about to beat the shit out of me? Or maybe they'd done something to my car; slashed the tyres, messed with the brakes. Maybe even planted a bomb.

I rushed out of there, back to the car, where Tony lay groaning on the passenger seat, puke on the gutter beside him. 'Greened out,' he mumbled, the term for too much pot, or for combining too much alcohol with pot.

I could have kissed him in gratitude. He'd sensed the threat too, and waited here to protect the car. We headed home to safety.

It wasn't possible to get used to the idea of a television speaking to me personally, not possible to ignore it. Worst of all, it was not possible to turn away, to *not* watch. It was as fascinating as it was terrifying. What confuses me to this day is: why didn't I reflect on the fact that this never *used* to happen? Why no signals before that period? Surely something had changed? I didn't ask myself those questions and I'm not sure why.

I spoke to no one about any of this. To do so seemed far too dangerous. Besides, it seemed everyone else must know. The signals were so obvious it was hard to believe others weren't aware of them, and everyone carried on as though this was nothing out of the ordinary. Radio and song lyrics also spoke to me personally. Often the signals were threatening, but just as often they seemed to convey approval, or to drop hints that great things awaited me. I was to be a rock star, Jim Morrison reincarnated, even Jesus. But I had to listen, decipher, and follow the signals. It was an impossible task; there were no frames of reference. Whose side was I on? The left wing or the right? Woolworths, Coke, Channel Nine?

People's words soon became a jumble of meaning nearly impossible to understand. Something as simple as 'Hey pass the butter, please' suddenly meant half a dozen different things at once, often as not with threats thrown in. I would answer them in the same language, with sentences which appeared normal on the surface but had multiple other meanings. I assumed everyone in the room was conversing on that hidden level with me, so bending the real-life relevance of what I said made little difference. The first hints of something amiss may have come when my responses to normal conversation became slightly abstract.

I visited Lisa every other day, utterly convinced that Woolworths had hired her. She only appeared after I started working for them, after all. Woolworths was no mere supermarket company; they had connections to other powerful entities — maybe the government, maybe the TV networks. Did they view me as such a potential asset that they would even hook me up with a partner in order to steer me in the right direction for the company? I was a supremely important being, after all, especially given that I was being sent all these signals, especially since I had the power to perceive it all, the ability to *just know* so many things. Still, was Lisa telling them personal things? Could I trust her? I had to be careful what I said around her.

From her perspective, I'd have seemed slightly eccentric, but then I'd been eccentric in high school, too. I was believing my Jim Morrison fantasy, and she bought into it a little, too. Paul had noticed intense hostility directed his way, thanks to my misinterpretation of his song lyrics, but that aside, there were few clues that anything was seriously wrong.

I began worrying about right-wing extremists, a fear sparked by a conversation I'd had during a visit to Lisa's relatives. That same night, *A Current Affair* did a story on the Ku Klux Klan, which neatly affirmed my concerns. The host, Mike Munro, offered his personal reassurance. His manner suggested I was being a little silly to worry so much. *We're on top of things*, he seemed to say.

The illness doesn't need such explicit connections to reality to convince the psychotic that something's up, but such things *do* affirm the delusions, and in any given twenty-four hour period, some kind of coincidence is almost inevitable; God forbid a day when there are two or three big ones lined up in a row. Suppose I make a cup of tea and a commercial for Tetley Tea comes on the television — *Aha! They're watching!* But suppose it's something completely unrelated — a commercial for Harvey Norman, say; the psychotic may discern some note of threat in the voiceover, apply it to an event of the day — tailgating that guy on the highway — and it's just as convincing.

The signals started coming from the radio, from advertisement billboards, from car licence plates, from newspaper headlines. DPU 632 on the car ahead of me suddenly meant Don't Push Us. Signals everywhere. Keeping track of them was fast becoming exhausting. And I just kept on smoking that weed.

FIVE

I was doing some casual work at a place that imported incense and statues of Indian gods. I was certain drugs and weapons were concealed in the shipments. I was on a smoke break out the front of the warehouse with Doug, Paul's friend. We'd been mucking around with cockney accents. My parked car was just in front of us. He asked me about the car's stereo; Brad and I had built two big ugly wooden speaker boxes, visible through the back windscreen. 'The speakers aren't working,' I told him.

'Probably got a wire loose,' said Doug. 'You should fiddle around with the wires.'

I nodded my understanding; he was warning me about the bug planted there to spy on me. I'd been aware of it for a little while now — it tracked my movements, listened in on my conversations. I'd figured it was better they think I didn't know it was there, yet Doug was saying I should disable it.

Chris, the boss, called me in to do a delivery. 'Just sign this form and take it to the post office,' he said. I took the package, but couldn't sign the form. I would be incriminating myself. The parcel was full of drugs; I'd be arrested. That was why he was getting *me* to deliver it, instead of taking it himself. I stood in his office, undecided.

'What's the problem?' Chris said.

'I don't know my way to the post office,' I said.

He gave me directions to the post office two streets away. Still I refused to sign the form.

Chris looked at me. 'Mate. What is the *problem*?'

I signed the form with a fake name, dropped it off at the post office, looking over my shoulder the whole time, searching for undercover agents. I spotted a couple — they looked just like regular people. Heads seemed to turn my way as I drove past in the boss's van.

When I got back to the warehouse, I apologised for refusing to sign the form. 'I don't sign something without knowing exactly what I'm signing,' I explained to Chris.

He gave me a funny look, but said not to worry about it.

It was closing time. I did a quick search in the front of my car, looking for the bug planted there. There might be cameras too. They were too well hidden to find.

Doug invited me back to his place for drinks. I declined, because Paul was going to be there. Paul was still the enemy. On the way home I took a big detour to throw off the people tracking me. I parked for a few minutes outside a building to confuse them and took twice as long to get home as normal. While I drove I sang songs — maybe whoever was listening in was a record executive or something. Or someone with music industry connections. Everyone had connections. Too many connections. Woolworths ... Coke ... television ... Lisa ... Paul ... Doug ... too many.

My war with Paul reached a climax one morning. I'd been unable to sleep the night before, I was so worked up. I'd read some new songs of his, such blatant potshots that I couldn't stand it. At about 3 am I wrote an angry letter, blaming him for imagined grievances, pledging never to forgive. I barged into his room, turned on the light, dumped the letter on his bed, and left him to try and make sense of it.

When morning came I heard him getting ready for work. I had to get away, leave the house until he was gone. I passed him in the hall. Without thinking I reached over and grabbed the front of his shirt, then restrained myself, let go, kept walking. Behind me, he muttered something. I didn't hear it, had no idea what he'd said, but it was enough. I turned back to him, threw a punch, and connected.

Justin shouted something and started trying to pull us apart. Mum was there fast, standing between Paul and me, separating us. Paul was looking bewildered, shaking his head, wondering what the hell had come over me. He left for work while Mum tried to find out what was wrong, what happened. I broke down, lying on the floor, saying something about reconciliation, reconciliation. My whole situation was the same as native Australia's, I told her. She didn't understand, no one did.

At the Indian import place, another frantic, confusing day passed. A few of us had been called in to unload a shipment. The other guys were friends of Paul's, and I knew he'd told them about how I'd struck him. They were distant and I was mortified.

Towards the end of the day, Chris asked me to fix up some of the shelves in the back of the warehouse. I was never good with tools and had to get another guy, Daniel, to help me out. He did most of the work; I was no help. 'Didn't your father ever teach you any of this stuff?' he muttered. A small remark, but it would become a big one. That sentence would reverberate inside and change the illness's script.

At closing time the other guys made plans for the night. They didn't ask me along. I hadn't driven to work today, so I walked across the city to the train station alone through crowds of people. Most of them looked at me like they recognised me. I stared straight ahead, trying not to look back. The city around me seemed like a concrete desert, lifeless, people blowing across it like tumbleweed.

Outside the train station I sat on the corner, smoking a cigarette. My head seemed suddenly empty of the rush of frantic thoughts that had been hurtling through all day, like I'd run out of fuel. Nothing added up anymore. The world around me was a mass of connections and hidden truths. And Daniel's remark replayed in my head, with its many layers of meaning: *Didn't your father ever teach you any of this stuff?*

A scrawny, weedy guy with dirty hair and a beard approached me. 'You need anything?' he asked. 'Whiz? Hammer?'

'Ah, man, I'm not a junkie,' I said in a resigned, sad way. 'I'm just a lost soul.'

'You sure you don't need anything?'

'You got any pot?'

He screwed up his nose in distaste. 'Nah, ain't got pot.'

I reached out and shook his hand like he was an old friend.

'Remember if you need anything, come see me,' he said as he walked away.

I walked through the station, and saw a security guard over my shoulder, watching me. Broken half-formed thoughts of systematic oppression and police states rattled through me. Arms raised, I walked up to him, asking incoherently why they couldn't just leave me alone. He said nothing, just watched me carefully, one hand on his radio. Waiting on the train platform, my brain started up again with renewed energy, like a machine spinning out of control, about Paul, about Dad.

The train came, full of football fans dressed in maroon. I dimly realised it was State of Origin night. A year ago I was knocking back beers at a friend's place, watching the game. Now I was living the novel *1984*. There was no freedom, there were cameras in televisions and everywhere else, watching everything we did. It was all real, Big Brother was watching *me*.

The swarm of football fans, yelling and braying, piled out of the train. I was a wreck when I got home. My mother saw I was a wreck, but still she didn't know why.

Dad, I soon realised, was the most dangerous person I knew. He had turned Paul and me against each other. I made a list of all the ills and misdeeds he'd committed against me. He was one of Them. My song lyrics had been trying to warn me all along. Reading through them, I was astonished not to have picked up on it before.

When he brought home some takeaway for dinner the next night, I knew better than to eat my share. He'd poisoned it. Mum watched as I examined my plate of food then pushed it away untouched. Her face showed worry. I didn't know what to make of it.

I left for work at Woolworths that same night. Dad had been in the shed, near my car. Before I started it, I spent ten minutes searching underneath it for a bomb he'd planted.

I patched things up with Paul as best I could, but I could no longer sleep when my father was in the house. My door didn't have a lock, and I could envision him creeping in during the night to kill me. The way he acted, feigning normality, was all the proof I needed.

One night I was desperate for sleep. My mind had been through so much unrest that I *had* to shut it down for a few hours. I grabbed Paul's and my books of lyrics, suspecting Dad would steal them for his own devices, then drove to the train station car park. I sat in the driver's seat, trying to sleep. It was deserted, silent and lonely. The sense of being watched was very real even here. Maybe there would be hit men on their way to the house; maybe my hidden allies had arranged Dad's death to protect me. A car passed on the road, heading towards our house. Did I really want them to kill my father? It was a hard question to answer. I couldn't knowingly let it happen, despite what I knew about him.

I drove home, not knowing what to do. I pulled into the driveway. The passing car hadn't come here. Was I disappointed? Maybe I *had* wanted the hit man to help. I blasted the horn several times into the still night, revved the engine and took off for Lisa's place. She was no longer in the caravan park — she'd moved into a rented house with a friend. Not wanting to wake her, I slept in the car outside.

Next morning she saw me there when she left for work. I explained that something was going on between me and Dad, and I couldn't sleep at home. I could not tell her exactly what was going on; it wasn't safe to, not without knowing how Woolworths would react. I had to drop hints and be oblique.

'You should have come in,' she said, concerned. She said I could stay at her place for a few days.

Dad was home when I returned to pick up some belongings. I couldn't find my book of lyrics and accused him of taking them. He was baffled. I suspected he might turn violent, so I grabbed a pair of scissors from the kitchen and stuck them in my pocket.

When I got to Lisa's, she wasn't home. Her mother sat in the lounge room, watching television. My eyes were red and watery. I tried to clean myself up a little. We chatted. She seemed to be warning me not to hurt her daughter, veiled in pleasantries and small talk. I took umbrage at the very idea, and veiled this reaction in pleasantries and small talk.

When she left, I saw the scissors were still sticking out of my back pocket. Maybe she'd seen them.

I sat in front of the television, waiting for Lisa to get home, trying to understand the signals that poured from the box in a steady stream.

SIX

Things had escalated to a point where my psychosis was now quite visible from the outside. Lisa began to see it, though she didn't know what it was. Paul had seen it for some time, my parents likewise, although up until now it had seemed to them to be just a teenage attitude problem.

Punching Paul was my only actual act of violence throughout this period, but to be honest I don't know what might have happened if I'd been left to the whims of psychosis for much longer. A person disposed towards violence is going to be much more dangerous, if psychotic. I am not that way disposed, but I was as scared as hell, and scared people can be dangerous. What if the security guard had seemed an imminent threat, back at the train station? I think of the scissors in my back pocket that afternoon and about what else could have happened, had my father come near me.

Memories become somewhat sketchy here; I don't recall a lot of specifics. I was hardly able to understand the language anymore, lost in a dozen interpretations of one simple sentence. One night my mother gave up trying to reason with me. I said something bleak and felt quite ready to give up and cut my wrists. She was in tears when she begged me to take a sleeping tablet and come with her to the doctor in the morning. It was, I think, a few days since I'd slept. My mother seemed one of the few in the world I could trust. I took the tablet and slept in Justin's room. His door had a lock on it.

Sleep helps. Somewhat calmer, I had a coffee and Mum drove me to the local GP. I chatted to him, but I wasn't saying much. I said, 'I think my dad is the problem ...' He asked me to elaborate but I refused. The doctor told me he remembered seeing me not so long ago, and that I'd seemed to be in a very different state of mind then. He recommended I see a psychiatrist and made the appointment for us.

A little later, we went to the nearest mental health clinic. I had an air of surrender about me. They were planning to put me to sleep like an animal for all I knew. My one hope was that someone would answer the riddles before they did it, explain all these connections, point out what was linked to what and to who; having those answers would be sweeter than anything else that could happen, any reward they could give me. Then it would be over.

In the waiting room there was a mirror in the high corner of the room. I looked sourly at the camera inside it while the psychiatrist spoke to my mum. Then she called me in and asked some questions. I calmly explained to her that there was no insanity, just a super-sanity. She asked me to repeat that and I did. I told her I knew she worked for the Inner Party (a reference to Orwell's *1984*) — that it was OK, I knew. She nodded and called in another doctor.

I told the second doctor some cryptic nonsense. He told me I was undergoing a drug-induced psychosis. He may as well have been speaking in Russian. With no will left to argue, I agreed to try the medication he prescribed. It was ten milligrams of Triazine, an antipsychotic. The female psychiatrist asked me if I understood what the medication was for.

'I've got a theory,' I told her.

'Well let's try an experiment,' she said, a little irritated.

I took one of the round white pills on the spot. Had I not agreed to take them I'd have been kept as an involuntary patient.

* * *

Triazine and I were destined to have a love-hate relationship, hate wearing the pants. The pills worked — I believe the expression is 'using a sledgehammer to crack a nut'. Almost immediately my thoughts slowed down, I became brain dazed and lethargic. Antispychotic meds are 'dopamine inhibitors', which means they basically deaden the part of the brain found to be overstimulated in psychotic minds. It's not a delicate operation, nor a precise one, but right now it's all we have.

The pills are serious, like being thumped nightly in the head with a brick. I felt lobotomised and simply didn't care about anything. Eighteen hours of sleep at a stretch was not uncommon. I read the pamphlets that came with the box of Triazine, but didn't understand a word.

My desire to get up in the morning, or do anything at all, dissipated. I was told these were 'negative symptoms' of the illness, but it seemed side effects from medication played no small part. I put on about twenty-five kilograms in a month, went from an athlete's body to being just some overweight guy. I was covered in stretch marks; belly, arms, upper thighs. I still have stretch marks from the amazing weight gain. When you sober up a little, that doesn't do wonders for your self-esteem. Over time I joined a few gyms, went for daily walks, arranged exercise schedules, tried to watch what I ate. Nothing worked while taking those fucking pills. I even tried to induce bulimia, but could never manage to make myself puke, no matter how far I rammed my fingers down my throat. I seriously contemplated liposuction. Mum talked me out of looking into it further.

It got harder to have sex as my libido became soft and timid, another side effect. I walked around in a stupor, though I still went to work at Woolworths (who were, it must be said, fantastic for their patience and understanding). I still smoked pot for a little while after diagnosis, failing to connect the drug to 'what had happened', but the meds were kicking in; in a way I could feel the wrestle between marijuana and Triazine. When I'd understood that marijuana was at least part of the reason for having to take these horrible meds, it was not hard to quit the dope.

Lisa exited stage left at some point, which was not an unreasonable decision, given what her boyfriend was becoming. At the time I didn't really care, hardly noticed. My emotions were dulled, another side effect. In those numb months I was nowhere near making sense of anything, coming to terms with anything. I still didn't know what the hell had hit me, only that it had knocked me over pretty convincingly, and that some things had changed for good.

In the meantime, eat, sleep, smoke. Consistency, stability, order.

I had no desire to do a thing or see anyone. Andrew did his best, trying to lure me out for a social game of tennis or cricket practice at the nets, but I wasn't interested. Symptoms still occurred, and I was trying to reconcile them with a mind which was gradually becoming more rational. Television was hard to watch, as signals still came. Long afterwards — I mean for *years* — signals still came. With time, they reduced in frequency and power. I watched old shows we'd taped years before and found signals in those old commercials, which confused me; these tapes were years old, how were they keeping up with current events?

Medication does only part of the job, albeit the most important part. The rest we must do ourselves: work through thinking processes, rebuilding a finely made structure of many delicate parts, intricately linked. It's slow going. My fear throughout this time was hearing voices. It hadn't happened yet, but doctors repeatedly asked me if I heard them. At night, the sound of a dog barking was enough to get me up, heart racing, wondering if this was the beginning of the dreaded voices. This fear was what kept me on the pills.

I began to let go of the rock-star fantasy I'd harboured. It was surprisingly hard to shake that off, even when there were fewer signals egging me on, even when I understood I had no talent for music, that it would never happen. It wasn't so much the illness that made it hard to shake off; I needed the sense of purpose that came from having something to strive for. I'd dragged myself along to band auditions, checked out local music magazines for people seeking vocalists, hung around guitar shops, penned songs. Now, with my confidence sapped due to weight gain, I no longer had the will to go through with it. One day, the thought just came to me: *Why not try writing?* You could do it at home, needed no expensive equipment, needed to pass no auditions.

Writing *had* occurred to me, not long before the psychotic episode. I'd had an idea for a fantasy story — a typical elves-and-wizards scenario — and had even made some notes in an exercise book. Then drugs and rock-star fantasies had taken over.

I bought a cheap ex-government computer, a piece of crap good for no more than word processing, then hit the second-hand book stores, loading up on Stephen King paperbacks. I reasoned I'd need to read a lot if I was serious about writing, so at first I didn't even do any writing, I just read for a couple of weeks.

When I started writing short stories, I was oblivious to the fact that none were particularly good; had I known they were not very good, I may not have kept at it. But they were coherent, whole pieces, with beginnings, middles and ends. Some stories showed promise; a story might have a decent ending, or a funny passage of dialogue, even if the overall result wasn't so hot.

My parents were delighted so see me doing something vaguely productive. I sometimes showed them the results. They were all smiles and encouragement, though I don't know if anyone took this endeavour for serious ambition just yet. I was serious as could be, but had no idea at all what I was in for, nor how much work was yet to be done.

A couple of months into it, I produced my first decent story: 'Chasing the Dragon'. In it, some kids are stoned on a newly discovered psychedelic drug, wandering through a field by the highway at night, when they come across a dragon. They're struck by its savage beauty, majestic size. One of them reaches out to touch it. It allows him to pet it, then dips its head down, inviting him to hop on for a ride. He's whooping and hollering as it lifts him high above the ground, then it tosses him into the air and bites him in half. The other stoned kids run away screaming.

STRANGE PLACES

Dad finished reading it and, excited, ran through the house looking for me. 'This is good!' he said, surprised and delighted. He hadn't been insincere the other times he'd praised my work, but I could tell he really meant it this time.

So I stuck at it. After all, there were long days full of time to kill and television was still too frightening to watch. What's more, it suddenly didn't seem like there was a hell of a lot to lose by taking a gamble with my life and chasing some kind of dream.

SEVEN

I re-enrolled in university, a Bachelor of Arts degree this time. (The idea of studying law in my medicated, confused state was fine comedy indeed.)

Being on campus around so many people was frightening; I did not handle crowds well, since the episode. Worse still was the work which required analysis of texts. It meant reading meaning into things like ads, films, articles — something which I'd proven to be a little too adept at over the last year, and had been quietly trying to remove from my general thought processes. I'd resolved that hints were now forbidden: someone could tell me something in plain language, black and white, or I'd ignore it. It would not have made for interesting flirting ...

Things with Paul and my father settled down when we all understood there had been a medical reason behind the recent drama. Dad no longer seemed to present any kind of danger, although there were moments here and there when I'd find extra meanings in some comment or other, an echo of the darker days before.

There was no major cognitive meltdown during this re-emergence into the world everyone else lived in, just lots of small ones. For example, I saw someone hurriedly leaving the university library with a floppy disk in his hand. There was something secretive about the way he hustled along the covered walkways; it suggested this disk contained my government file or something. I followed him halfway across the campus to see where he was headed with my information, but lost sight of him.

Those smaller incidents were like biting mosquitoes, easily waved away, but plentiful. But their existence made it possible to believe that there *was* still some giant hidden world, just out of sight. You're not quite able to trust which perceptions are real and which are delusional. Would an advertising company spend hundreds of thousands of dollars on a television commercial — from a bunch of ad execs brainstorming around a table for ideas, to shooting it (hair, make-up, lighting), to the edit, to buying air time for the campaign, making sure it was screened during a show they knew I'd be watching — for the sole purpose of freaking me out or sending some message of approval or warning? It's easier now to see that it's absurd than it was back then; back then, TV seemed like some kind of witchcraft, just those pictures and sounds coming out of a box. And even today, if I skipped medication for a while and smoked a joint, maybe it wouldn't seem absurd anymore.

Was life on track again? Was that possible, so soon? I was twenty, passing at uni, I'd decided to be a writer (not knowing yet what that decision really meant). On track or not, the direction I was travelling in had changed. But there was no happily ever after yet. I was heavier, unfit, smoked thirty cigarettes a day at least. I felt dumber. And because I felt dumber, I began to mess around with the medication. I wanted to write, and being dumbed down wouldn't help that one little bit. To compensate for the feeling of medicated lethargy I drank lots of coffee. I stayed up for longer periods of time, sometimes forgoing sleep for twenty-four hours and hence prolonging the time between doses of Triazine.

My parents kept an eye on me, though, and I wasn't able to skip medication for long. It was an occasional protest against the side effects of the pills. I did it to feel smarter, like my old self. Then I'd see something on television, pick up a signal, panic, rush back to the pills, sleep for incredibly long stretches of time, and count down the time before I could come off the medication for good.

A doctor told me it might take three years or so before that could happen. A little white lie told for my own good.

Months passed sluggishly. I saw a psychiatrist once a month or so, for checkups. These meetings rarely lasted more than a few minutes — their job seems to end once they've found the best dose of medicine for you. They asked irritating questions, like 'How are your thoughts?' I ran out of original ways to answer this. The doctors invariably asked if I was still smoking pot. They asked if I was using speed. They kept on asking, and I didn't understand the reason at the time: to see if the diagnosis of drug-induced psychosis was correct, or if it was actually something more permanent. Drug-induced psychosis goes away when the drug use ceases. They didn't seem to believe me when I told them I'd quit the drugs.

I asked them what the medication was doing to me, and never got an answer I could understand. I was told vague things like: 'It will keep your thoughts on track.' I didn't want to hear that, I wanted to know exactly what the chemicals in the pills were doing. Eventually I was told something about a 'chemical imbalance' in my brain that these meds were correcting. That still seemed vague. I got the feeling the doctors didn't know very much about it themselves, that their job was just to dispense pills and ask annoying questions.

Every week I saw a case worker. Case workers are not doctors — their job is to keep an eye on you, offer a shoulder to lean on, write up 'plans' and 'goals' for you, all that sort of shit. My case worker told me that psychosis, once experienced, goes one of three ways. For one third of people, it's a one-off thing, never a problem again. For another third of people, they experience the problem again once or twice in their lives. For the final third of people, it becomes a permanent problem, lifelong.

Still, I could never trust that medication. I kept thinking that the side effects were deliberately put in there, so we'd get depressed and then need to buy antidepressants manufactured by the same pharmaceutical company that made the antipsychotics. Or maybe the side effects were some sort of deliberate ideological punishment for 'knowing too much'. Neither seems especially likely now in the cold light of sanity. That they were a pain in the arse, however, is indisputable.

For a time, six or seven months, I was pretty much on top of things. Having accepted the goal of a three-year endurance of pills, it was time to grit my teeth and bear the side effects of Triazine. Uni was easy enough and I kept writing stories. I even moved out of home with Andrew and a fellow called Nathan, an old school chum

I'd bumped into at uni. Nathan was very short, very smart, slightly elfish-looking and had long silky black hair — his pride and joy — which was thinning at a merciless rate.

We found a rental house — not easy to do given real-estate agents' paranoia about alcohol-friendly young men with no rental history — and managed to find some hand-me-down furniture. Each of us chipped in a hundred bucks for a second-hand fridge. We grew accustomed to each other's mess, to Nathan's beautiful long black hair weaving its way into the carpet, and discovered the joys of packet pasta and bourbon on Wednesday nights, the way only bachelors can.

I kept writing stories and honing the craft, but progress was slow. 'Editing' to me then meant barely more than running a spell-checker. It was a phase of psychological barriers being overcome — first, writing a story of more than three thousand words. For some reason, nearly every story was around the three thousand word mark, each written in one sitting. Silly as it sounds, it was a big deal the first time I stopped a story, left it overnight, then came back to it the next day to finish it off. Though a couple of stories showed signs of branching out, they were mostly horror stories at this point, as horror was pretty much all I read. One nasty little story I showed Nathan disturbed him so much he seriously considered moving out. (Actually, it was the kind of story you'd have trouble taking seriously unless the author was in the next room while you were asleep.) I was still years away from writing anything publishable, but some of those earlier works might have come reasonably close, had they been properly rewritten and edited.

The prospect of writing a novel — or even a novella of, say, thirty thousand words — was far beyond me. I had no idea how to go about it, though I made hesitant attempts in an exercise book, thinking that writing longhand would somehow crack the secret. How the hell did you squeeze that many words out of a single idea?

Meanwhile, it kept gnawing at me that the pills were making me stupider, that I could write much better if I stopped taking them. The stories I wrote when I'd skipped the medication for a while seemed to read much better. I'd have a week off the meds here and there, perhaps taking a tablet once every couple of days. I stopped seeing psychiatrists. I didn't want a case worker, with their 'plans' and jargon about 'stressors' and self esteem-building; talking to them, and to doctors, made me feel more ill than ever, reminding me of all the symptoms I was trying to put behind me. (It's strange that even today it still feels that way, a little ... You forget about 'the condition' until it's time to talk to a doctor about it, and it takes you right back to those moments when you were just put on medication for the first time.) I kept the medication handy, ready to use if I felt really bad on a particular day. But the side effects weren't worth it.

And so I began to fight against the illness without medical aid. I lost five kilos very quickly with minimal effort. Getting to sleep unaided was the hard part. We were also drinking heavily on a regular basis, which was not a great investment in mental health, not least because of alcohol's depressant effect. Alcohol's also capable of triggering symptoms if it's overdone, especially to those who should be on meds but aren't. And we overdid it.

One time I recall vividly. I'd been taking a break from writing, watching television. It had been gnawing at me for a while that I should get back to work. An ad for some headache tablet or other came on, and the phrase that got me was: '... HARD WORKING medicine'. It was an instruction to get back to my room and write, explicitly tailored to my circumstances.

If They were giving me an order, this meant They were watching me, which meant I was exceptionally important, and They had great, grand plans for me. I'd convinced myself *some* of the past delusions were just that, delusions; but how much of it was real? *Some* of it had to be, at least.

You couldn't tell me *every* little part of it was a mirage. Which parts weren't?

To test myself, I sat in front of the news each night, waiting for more signals. Because I was looking for signals, I started finding them. There was a report of a 'home invasion', three streets away from our house. The bandits had carried shotguns but not fired them. The distraught family on camera said, 'Maybe they'll use the guns next time!' This was clearly a direct threat. They'd hired thugs to terrorise a family, just to scare me. What had I done to offend them? Was it something I'd written? How had they seen what I'd written? I'd hardly shown anyone the stories.

The old questions began again: *How do they know I'm watching right now? Can they see me this very moment? Well, where's the camera?* Every night was terrifying, but I kept watching the news, afraid that I'd miss something vital for survival. I didn't start taking the tablets again.

It was a hard battle. Sometimes, locked in my room at night, unable to sleep, my mind felt like a war zone. I pictured a pair of train tracks, a single cart full of my thoughts, rocketing downhill at an increasing pace, wobbling and speeding, in imminent danger of spilling its cargo all over the tracks as it derailed. When it sped down the hill too fast, rocking from side to side, I'd take a once-off dose of medication, and it would be like a metal clamp coming down on top of the cart, slowing it, steadying. Stop the pills, the clamp releases, and again the cart plunges forward, slowly at first ...

Some days passed in relative peace, usually the days I stayed away from TV. This made me believe that the illness could really be beaten, that it was just a matter of letting time pass and riding out the rough patches, that my mind would inevitably heal like a physical injury.

Nice idea, but I was growing unstable. When we drove to uni Andrew noticed me asking if certain cars were following us. At one time, I suspected that Andrew was going to get even for that party we'd thrown at his parents' house a couple of years before, or for some imagined wrongs, and kill me. For a brief period, I was genuinely afraid of him, once refusing to get in the car with him for fear he'd crash on purpose to kill us both.

I assumed I was being watched. Occasionally I'd hear on TV a phrase I'd used in a story and freak out. I found myself, almost without thinking, checking my room for cameras. I stuck dark tape over a few holes in the plaster that looked suspicious. Then I would tell myself to calm down, to relax, that *I was not so important that anyone would want to bother monitoring me.*

I spoke to no one about all of this. This time, there weren't many obvious clues for others to pick up on, unless they had the trained eye of a psychiatrist. Avoiding the pills was my main concern, which necessitated camouflage.

Then, strangely, things seemed to settle down into some sort of remission. Still without the medication, I began to improve, found sleep easier to come by. What brought this change about I can't say, but I was pretty certain that I had the illness licked. It was now a thing of the past and I began to think of it as 'that thing that happened a while back'. But the battle had tired me a great deal. And the reprieve was temporary, as it turned out.

Andrew moved out because we were suddenly at each other's throats. Our new roommate was another friend from high school, Robert. He was a big guy, with white curly hair and glasses, and an almost constant Cheshire cat grin, which could freak you out if you didn't know him. He spoke in a quiet, slow voice, which had a soothing effect on me, handy especially on more turbulent days of mental turmoil. We became pretty good friends.

He and Nathan were another matter. Robert, for all his apparent placidity, had a flash-flood temper, and he was a large fellow — you could pick better enemies. Once, at Nathan's old place, there'd been an incident. Nathan and some of his friends went out on a house-egging spree and, finding Robert's car parked by the road with the driver's side window down, they'd succumbed to temptation. In response, Robert went slightly crazy, throwing chairs at the windows of the house, a genuine rampage. It took six guys to hold him back. Some animosity remained between Robert and Nathan. When Nathan was offered another place to live, he took it.

Another of the high school chums moved in, a guy named Trent. He was not dissimilar to Robert; a heavyset guy with glasses, a goatee, and a quiet, speak-only-when-spoken-to manner. It was hard to pry either of them away from their computers, which they set up in the living room in a nest of wires and cords. Not strictly life in the fast lane, more like life in a cocoon, neatly cut off from the real world. But it was comfortable.

For a while, anyway.

EIGHT

It's strange. The time Dawn spent with us couldn't have been more than a few weeks, two months tops, but in my memory it seems to take up a large portion of space. In part I guess it's because this was the time of the engine trouble that came before I nosedived towards full-blown insanity again. I remember it so vividly, this time before the big crash.

The computer networks and pay TV at our house were like a bachelor magnet. (Pay TV being a luxury Trent and Robert had decided we could not live without. My eyes spent more time on the portable unit's red light — is that a camera? — than on the screen.) You could leave KFC wrappers everywhere and no one would hassle you; you could drink bourbon at any time of day and not be judged. Hence, a bunch of guys we'd hung around with at school — not the army guys; a more library-oriented group — were prone to drop in. One of them, Louis, made our place his home away from home. Louis was six foot two with long black hair, and looked like he'd spent a lot of time around guitars, although he hadn't. Louis had probably the highest IQ out of anyone I knew. He was enrolled in a science degree at my uni, but spent most of his time at our place watching movies and making wisecracks at whatever was on TV.

Louis started a fling with a girl from Melbourne, Dawn, via EverQuest, the online role-play computer game which all of us played at the time. In the game, thousands of players interact in a virtual fantasy world, completing quests and hunting monsters and so on. It was the presence of this hideously addictive game in our home that saw writing gradually fall off my radar. Whenever Robert was out, I'd hop on his computer and tromp around in an actual fantasy world as a dark elf necromancer. More fun than writing; easier, too. Anyway, Louis's barbarian warrior got to chatting with a foxy dark elf cleric, and they got on well, despite the race/class difference.

Online relationships occur under slightly false pretences; with time to think before you speak, it's easier to be witty and charming, and the delete button is a godsend. With this advantage, Louis charmed Dawn for a couple of weeks, and she invited him to come and visit her in Melbourne. He would spend a week at her sharehouse, then she would come to Brisbane.

So down he went, Louis's first real contact with womankind. Robert and I chatted online with them, helping ease their evident tension. When Louis wasn't around, Dawn would tell me they weren't getting along, listing his various defects. In a sick way I was delighted to hear it all; why should Louis get action when the rest of us were doomed not to? They had soon had enough of each other and Louis made plans to head back home. But Dawn still intended to come up to Brisbane. She wanted to meet the rest of us. With the delete key, and that extra couple of seconds to type out responses in conversations, we seemed sophisticated, witty and mysterious.

I hadn't had female company since Lisa. In our four-way chats online, I began to realise that I was trying to win Dawn over, though it was more a game than actual ambition. To have her physically *here*? I never counted on that. Life was simple, dull and safe now: pay TV, junk food, computer games, extended adolescence. I looked at myself in the mirror: some improvement, but still overweight. The stretch marks were still visible. Her arrival began to loom in my mind like some coming biblical cataclysm, anticipated with awe and dread.

STRANGE PLACES

There was a gym a couple of minutes' walk up the road. Robert and I joined. We had a week to shape up before she arrived.

In the beginning Dawn had a place lined up in Brisbane, and a job lined up too. As the date of her arrival drew closer, the place she'd lined up fell through. She asked if it would be OK to stay at our place. She could pay some rent, she said, until she found somewhere to live. The job was still lined up — until, of course, it also fell through. She'd no longer be able to pay some of the rent. Was that still cool?

Robert was fine with it. Trent was fine with it. None of us knew what she looked like yet, but our standards weren't high, and she fitted the main criterion: female. A definite step up. I voiced the only opposition. I asked the hard questions. Is she going to chip in for bills? How long will she be hanging around our house? Who *is* this chick anyway? What does she want from us?

My growing apprehension seemed to fuel some odd chemistry with Dawn when we chatted online. I was distrustful and pensive. This only seemed to encourage her. Had I declared my undying love, asked her what we'd name our first child, she'd have fled in a heartbeat.

The day finally came. Dawn and Louis arrived in Brisbane. The last few days I'd had a relapse back into the 'war zone' frame of mind, fighting off discordant thoughts, battling hard for sanity. Most of the fears were Dawn-related — who did she work for? Which secret organisation? — but there were some of the old demons returning too.

Robert and I drove to the airport to pick them up in separate cars. We got our first look at her by the luggage belt, where she and Louis were deep into a tense silence. At first glance she seemed older than she really was, but it was just tiredness from the flight north. Caught somewhere between hippie and punk, she wore a purplish-pink tie-dyed dress, had short black hair, a slim but curvaceous body, a pierced chin and tongue.

Robert and I said a quick 'hello' as we helped carry Dawn's luggage. She seemed amused by this chivalry. It was awkward — we'd all spoken for a while online, but no one had much to say in the flesh. She had a lot of stuff with her, including a laptop and her bass guitar. The bass intrigued me very much, and rock-star fantasies stirred again.

We headed back to the car, Dawn and Robert walking ahead of Louis and me. I asked him about his stay down there, eager to gather intelligence on where he and Dawn stood. 'I think it's official,' he said. 'We hate each other.' He told me about what they'd been up to in Melbourne, including many dark clubs and strip joints. I told him I thought she was a teensy bit unstable (ironic, eh?). He agreed without elaboration. I asked Louis if he thought the whole trip had been worthwhile. Was he glad he'd gone? How would he describe the whole experience?

'Expensive,' he muttered. Then he remarked somewhat cryptically: 'One man's trash is another's treasure.' Indeed.

Dawn is in a house full of girl-shy computer geeks. Robert calls a few more old library buddies to come around and break the ice. It helps a little. Everyone hangs out in the lounge room, trying to make our guest feel at home in the Sunshine State with one-liners, guffaws and *Simpsons* quotes. Meanwhile I'm slinking around in the background, chewing fingernails in anxiety, doing last minute push-ups, cursing the mirror.

They set up Dawn's computer in the living room; there will be much EverQuest played in the coming weeks. The hot potato issue of where she's going to sleep during her stay has not yet been raised. I know damned well the answer to that question. The notion is fucking me up, but it's inevitable.

Andrew came over late that afternoon. We decided to hit the town. A group of seven drove into the city in separate cars. Everything seemed a bit subdued. It was a weeknight so the city was quiet. We went to Doolies, a large pub/club with many pool tables. We found a table and chatted. Louis and Dawn's quiet animosity continued with little snide remarks and rolled eyes.

Beers were consumed. I stayed sober, chatted to Dawn a little. There was some low-key flirting, both ways. It was pretty obvious how things were going to pan out. It was indescribably awkward, almost saddening, similar to how I'd felt when going to the mental health clinic for the first time: let's get this over with. Back home, I would not say my performance sent shudders of disquiet through the ranks of male porn stars. No practice makes imperfect.

Lying there with a stranger in my bed made sleep impossible. My thoughts were speeding up. The cart on the tracks was rocking from side to side, speeding downhill. Its cargo was in danger. I got up, grabbed the packet of Triazine from my desk. It was buried under a pile of papers and notebooks, untouched for about five months. Dawn watched without saying anything, and there was something knowing in her silence — she had seen these kinds of pills before, had maybe guessed a thing or two about me into the bargain. I took one five-milligram tablet, half my prescribed dose, and washed it down. It was the last time I ever took the stuff.

* * *

The meds had spoken: I slept until mid-afternoon, then woke feeling groggy and clouded. Dawn and Robert had been getting acquainted while I was out of it — presumably by now his Cheshire cat grin had ceased being disconcerting to her. Louis was quietly hanging around the living room and gave me funny looks when I emerged. Trent had been lying low. I poured caffeine into my system to try and speed up the brain.

I had a chat to Dawn when the guys went out. She said she was a pagan, but the equivalent of a believer who doesn't go to church on Sundays anymore. While we talked her eyes seemed to be playing tricks. It looked like her irises were changing size, left then right, expanding then shrinking. It was hypnotic, though whether it was actually happening or just a trick of my haywire brain, I'm not sure to this day. Some conclusions could not be avoided: she had magic powers. This was intriguing and pleasantly scary. She seemed a little manic when we talked about certain subjects; her eyes would light up, her grin would look slightly evil as she stared off into space while she spoke.

Dawn and I weren't really an item. We stopped screwing on about the third day of her stay, once she judged her vengeance against Louis had been sufficiently wreaked. She was getting along well with Trent and Robert, but becoming a thorough enigma to me. One afternoon we were driving through the suburbs. I had started getting signals from outside sources again and I'd noticed a licence plate combination which I seemed to be seeing very frequently, all of a sudden. CVN 192. The numbers would vary, but the letters stayed constant. CVN, it meant something but there was no telling what. Were these secret government cars?

We were stopped at the lights. The car in front of us had a licence plate that read CVN 393. I looked at it then looked away, pretending not to notice anything; dismissing signals began with showing no outward sign that you'd heard or seen something amiss. If They didn't think you'd seen it, that signal would not become an ongoing dialogue; you could try to forget about it later.

In the passenger seat, Dawn turned to me and said, 'That's an interesting licence plate.' She studied my face for a reaction and probably saw one. She'd noticed the licence plates. She'd seen them too. She knew *I* could see them. This was a very big deal.

I was now on high alert whenever Dawn spoke. We were on our way to see a movie, *Charlie's Angels*. The theme of undercover female spies was not lost on me. Afterwards, as we walked through the car park, she told me that she'd wanted to be a writer, once. She said she'd written a play about a secret war between television and computers.

Poker face on, I chuckled, made some noncommittal flippant remark, but I was reeling inside. What she'd told me was a major hint — about herself, about the world. Whose side was she on in this great war? She was here to recruit me for one side or the other — TV or computers? So *those* were the two great sides, the grand fire spawning all these smoke signals I'd picked up since that first time in the living room at my parents' house.

They'd planned this revelation. People were watching us right now as we crossed the car park, studying my body language to see where my loyalties lay. There would be the passing or failing of some great secret test. Then my reward: someone would finally tell me the truth about the world, map all these connections out clearly. They'd use me to help win their war, and they'd grant me protection. Yes, Dawn's revelation was colossal, and it coloured a lot of the symptoms to come.

If this thinking wasn't actively psychotic already — to me it looks like it was — I was at the very least slipping. But when you're slipping you don't tend to realise it until you're on the other side, doped up on meds, a psychiatrist informing you it happened again.

On and on it went. It's more than possible I made her nervous, too. One morning she told me: 'Some people are dangerous because they have a reason to hurt other people. They're pissed off or something. But I don't need a reason. That's sort of scarier.'

No shit, Dawn. No shit.

An example of how language sounds in the ear of a psychotic ...

On a shopping trip, we stopped in at Acid Gear, a shop that does body piercing. Dawn had two pierced nipples, a pierced tongue and chin, and both ears were drilled. She ogled the spread of jewellery behind the glass case and chatted with the blonde behind the counter. Some tattooed guy came out from the back of the shop. I bristled for a moment or two as he checked Dawn out. Dawn, seemingly oblivious to this, told the woman behind the counter she might come back and have something done next week.

'Yeah, well at least you know what we've got now,' said the woman behind the counter.

They were talking about me. That tattooed guy walking past was another test, all prearranged. 'At least you know what we've got now,' meant: *So, he's the jealous type. At least he's got a pair.* This, in turn, meant: *He may come in useful, but that immature streak could be costly to our underground black magic network. Hopefully he'll grow out of it and be able to serve us better.* All this was interpreted in real time, on the spot, no time taken to think about it.

STRANGE PLACES

Dawn dared me to get a piercing. To her surprise, I said I would. She egged me on. 'Bill! Hard*core*!' Robert, my conservative roommate, asked me with unconscious irony if I was out of my mind. I told him of course not.

I chose the septum, thinking of the singer of the metal band Sevendust. Through a curtain was a back room with a dentist-style chair. A muscular middle-aged woman pulled on some rubber gloves and produced a huge needle. I closed my eyes as she poked it through the gap of skin between the bottom cartilage of my nose and the ridge of flesh between the nostrils, two individual punctures, one on each side. It hurt like hell. My eyes watered and it bled a little. I'd picked the ring that looked like a bull horn.

Back at the counter the delicate issue of payment was raised. I only had sixty bucks. It cost one hundred and twenty-five. The underground network was discovering that they wouldn't have the services of a breadwinner. Dawn had volunteered to pay as part of the dare, something I reminded her of now. 'I didn't think you'd actually do it though,' she protested. We split the cost before I had to bring up the issue of her rent-free existence. Robert kept looking at me like I'd just stuck a fork in a power socket. He hardly said a word on the way home.

The ring had a strange effect on me; it seemed to put me in charge of things a little more. I felt different now, hardcore. If Dawn was a witch, maybe I was a warlock in training. Meanwhile I was losing weight fast. Gym was a daily event and it was working.

People seemed to notice me more since the piercing. Once this would have filled me with terror, but now I didn't mind. It was invigorating — like a pre-episode high ...

NINE

Strange. Things calmed right down when Dawn returned to Melbourne. She'd grown sick of sleeping on the fold-out sofa bed, and I was sick of seeing her walk around the house in her underwear then behaving like a nun if I went near her. We were snappy with each other and our goodbyes weren't pleasant.

Louis and I bought a twenty-dollar bottle of bourbon the night she left. We couldn't work out if we were commiserating or celebrating her departure.

As the lazy summer break stretched out before me, things became close to normal again. Better than normal; things were great. I was in better shape than I'd ever been, visiting the gym every second day, swimming laps every day. Before long the smoking problem was licked too. It was surprisingly easy, though the last two quit attempts had been a nightmare. This time, a little pain in the kidneys from adjusting to toxin levels was the worst of it.

I could no longer understand my roommates, who found everything they wanted out of life in computer games and pay TV. I tried to tell them a world existed outside this living room but they didn't believe me.

By the time uni started again, life was going as well as it possibly could be. There seemed an aura of positive energy about me. I was confident as hell, bulletproof. Unfortunately, since I wasn't taking my medication, it was only a matter of time before all this would change — and not very much time at that.

Our university Orientation Week fell at the end of February. A bunch of clubs and activist groups had set up stalls and were passing out pamphlets to students. A stunning twenty-something woman from Greenpeace stepped in front of me as I walked past and said, 'Excuse me, would you like to help Greenpeace?'

There was something in the way she said it. Those words resonated — *help Greenpeace* — like a command while hypnotised. This was, I think, the moment the nosedive began; a couple of weeks later I'd crash-land in a mental ward. I looked into her eyes, thought for a second, then said 'Sure!' I signed their papers, pledged ten dollars a week to their cause. It felt like I was in a euphoric trance the whole while. The feeling remained for a minute or two as I walked away to my class. It felt, literally, that some kind of magic had been worked on me.

And of course it had been seen. People were watching me now, people on both sides of politics. They were out of sight, hidden in the crowds of students, but *watching*. Helping Greenpeace had been a public declaration of loyalty to the left. I wasn't scared this time — on the contrary, it felt good to know where battle lines were drawn, to pledge allegiance to one side. It meant enemies on campus, but also allies.

It meant someone needed to take his fucking pills.

As well as licence plates, TV and radio, I began picking up signals in body language in that first week back at uni. I watched people's hands when they spoke. If their thumb flicked upwards at any point, it was 'thumbs up', meaning I'd done or said (or thought) the right thing. I didn't examine the logic closely enough to see that this implied everyone could read my mind. When I took notes during lectures, I'd look up at the lecturer's hands for confirmation my notes were correct. It became a way to map out this new landscape of reality, in which I was a vital weapon in the hidden war.

I sat in a small lecture room as the teacher, a fifty-something academic who spoke like a preacher, showed us a video dramatisation of the Spanish Inquisition. 'They targeted leaders,' he said. His eyes were on me when he said this. It was a friendly warning, just so I knew what I'd be in for if I accepted my role as a 'chosen one'. *Well good*, I thought, vowing to be a martyr if necessary. *Target me.*

At home, signals from the television came nonstop. Now, though, things had changed since that first signal. I was no longer clueless: there was a war between TV and computers, somehow running alongside the war between the left and right wings of politics, of heaven and hell, good and evil. Every signal revealed a fraction more of the landscape, and of my hugely important role in this grand war.

There was an ad for Daikin air conditioners I found especially hard to watch. The ad was going on about how smart these air conditioners are: '... *Daikin KNOWS because Daikin air conditioners have a HIGHER INTELLIGENCE ...*'

It was terrifying to be openly taunted like this. I switched the channel, waiting for the ad to finish. I switched back a minute later, but the same ad was on again. '... *Because Daikin Air conditioners are going to murder you in your sleep, William ...*'

I could stand no more. 'Oh fuck your air conditioner,' I said to the screen. The television seemed to go silent. I sensed stunned people on the other end of the box — those hateful people whose job it was to read my reactions, to send their messages. Now they sat there unable to speak, knowing their power over me was gone. I could almost hear them saying, 'He's not afraid? What are we supposed to do now?' It felt like a victory. I was no longer afraid of the TV. I wanted to fight it.

My lecturer in Professional Ethics was, I concluded, one of the Enemy. I argued with almost everything he said. The other students began groaning whenever I raised my hand.

It was in the second week of study that things came to a head. I still have the notebook lying around:

> Public versus private morality: taking moral stance is a decision between fear and courage. Ethical imperative versus personal danger.

'It's difficult to take a public moral stance,' the lecturer said. 'Sometimes people come under personal threat ...'

A threat aimed at me. *Fine!* I thought, remembering I was willing to die.

As though he was reading my mind, the lecturer upped the ante. 'And then sometimes their *families* come under threat ...'

Son of a bitch, I thought, *he's the voice of the system. They'd stoop that low, would they? All the more reason to fight them* ... and on it went.

The cart tipped in that class, I think. Spilled all over the place. As the lecturer spoke, he kept glancing back at his podium. I suddenly realised why. There was a screen there. A camera was rigged over my right shoulder, up in the roof, and he was reading my notes.

I was scared for a second, then came a feeling of triumph, for here was my chance to tell Them that I knew *They* knew, and I didn't care, it didn't matter. Knowing the lecturer was reading, I started writing some notes.

Are you watching, you fat fuck?

He paused and stuttered mid-sentence. It was all the proof I needed. Time to send some signals of my own.

Buy me — I see both sides

He was checking the podium (screen) more often now, pausing to read what I'd written and trying to think fast to respond. Everything he said held threats and mockery. 'So, getting back to the point of *public* morality as separate from *private* morality…'

You want me on your team — trust me

'… who consider a moral position just a form of self-indulgence …'

But you don't have me on your team … YET

'… to consider marketing and sharing of personal information …'

Now you know my stance

' … to be a case of moral blindness…'

I'm not expensive. I cannot afford groceries. This is my stance.

'… the ethical imperative versus reasonableness…'

silence is GOLDEN

The class finished. I walked out of there victorious, and the look I shot my lecturer as I passed him showed it.

It may have been that same afternoon when, at home in my room, I began sketching in my notebook. I drew a picture of the Christian cross and was struck by a revelation. It struck me that the cross was the entire model of our society. Two arms — one left and one right — were the political arms. Then there were two arms going up and down. Left–right: the political. Up–down: the economic. All conflicting forces sat somewhere on this model: heaven/hell. Men/women. Television/computers.

It made perfect sense to my scrambled brain. Left and right, the only two viable ways of thought. Up and down, the emotions we feel. Like the economy, rising and falling. We're meant to *feel* on this up–down level, and to *think* on the left–right level. It seemed a huge revelation, of massive importance — the ultimate secret.

I thought again of bipolar and psychosis. The two travel along these planes. Psychosis spins, horizontally, left and right, like a cyclone. Bipolar wavers up and down, like the seasons of the year. Of course! I had uncovered the innermost bindings of the world. But now I was more dangerous to Them than ever, which made Them more dangerous to me.

I leaned back on my bed, stared up at the light in the ceiling for maybe fifteen minutes. Something that one of my lecturers had said came back to me. He'd turned on the fluorescent lights at the start of the class, and said jokingly, 'Let there be light. *Electric* light.'

Naturally. He'd been warning me. I knew I was looking into a camera but I kept staring. They'd been watching me the entire time. They'd seen everything I put into my notebooks. They'd seen everything, period. The sense of betrayal and grief was enormous.

I wrote some more notes, but in code this time. They may be able to see everything, but they weren't inside my head. Yet.

The weekend came. Andrew called one night and invited me to a party held by some people he worked with. Trent, my roommate, was playing a game on his computer nearby, and he thumped the table in frustration because his character died. I saw his fist clump down on the wood, a signal: *Don't go, there's a bunch of guys there who are going to beat you up.*

I trusted signals from Trent. I stayed home that night.

Back at uni, the Monday of week three. I was mulling over the up–down, left–right revelation. It was too important to keep to myself — the other students had to be shown. But it could not be said explicitly; that would put them at risk. I bought a can of soft drink, a symbol of the economy. As I walked to the lecture theatre, past a crowd of students having late breakfast or coffee, I opened the can and drank. With each step I tilted my head upward and guzzled a mouthful. Then I lowered my head, my chin on my chest, as though depressed, shuffling my feet slowly. Next step, raised my head again and drank another mouthful. Up–down my head went.

I must have looked ridiculous.

Outside the room of my lecture, people waiting for the class gave me funny looks as I walked past them. I tossed the can into the bin inside the room, sat down and felt like I'd achieved something important, scored points for my team, hurt the enemy.

I had removed the septum piercing some time ago to do a little casual work at the airport. But now, powerful signals had told me the importance of having the piercing back — it was how my allies would recognise me, and would warn enemies to keep their distance. I was alone in the house; Robert was at his new girlfriend's place, presumably still grinning like a Cheshire cat, and Trent was at work.

I'd spent much of the morning by the living-room window on sentry duty, peering out at the road. When a police car drove past, the terror was immense. I was an enemy of the state, and here they were, come to drive me out of hiding.

Robert's car was still in our driveway. He'd left his keys inside. I started up and drove off. The police car was parked two houses up the road. As I drove slowly past, the cop car crept forward a few metres, like a wolf stalking.

I drove away. I'd narrowly escaped the concentration camps, but they might still be following. I didn't know where to go, had to trust my intuition. I ended up at the Acid Gear shop, where I'd had the septum job done. My eyes were red when I got there, my hands visibly trembling. The girl behind the counter, the same one who'd been there when Dawn was with us, asked me what I'd like done. Her eyes were doing the same trick that I'd seen Dawn's do, the irises expanding and shrinking, left then right. Some sort of spell to placate me — she was afraid of me. The woman who did their piercings wasn't in at the moment; I was invited to wait around till she showed up. I sat on a couch inside the shop and read magazines, which instructed me on my role in the world that would come, once the revolution had done its work.

The burly woman showed up, took me into the back room. 'Why did you take the last one out?' she asked me.

'I had to for work.'

'That'd be right,' she said, shaking her head at whoever had asked me to do this. She seemed like a doctor patching up a wound others had maliciously inflicted. Her manner made me trust her completely. She produced a big needle and began the process of widening the gap in my septum. 'Come on now,' she said. 'I can feel you fighting me. We'll get it in there.'

I was fighting, too, backing away and fidgeting. I felt like a scared animal on a vet's operating table. This was something I had to do, not a choice. She stuck the needle into the existing hole, the right side first. The pain was intense.

I paid them and left, and somehow felt better, as though the woman's punctures had released some steam-valve of dangerous energy. Still not knowing where to go, I headed towards town and mulled over the words I'd hissed with each puncture: *Fuck! Jesus!* Did it mean I was Jesus, or the Antichrist, or some combination of both?

But the worst was over. The world had been about to close in — now it backed away.

Before long it became apparent I was headed for Paul's place in Carseldine. Was it wise to bring his home to the attention of those following me? Stopped at the lights, the passenger in the car ahead of me flicked his hand, which dangled outside the window — a gesture like someone swatting away a fly. *Go back.*

It was a clear signal, but I was still unsure. Another passenger's hand in a car further ahead gestured in the same way. *Go back.*

I turned down the street to Paul's place. Go back? Show them I'm not afraid? Maybe that's what was needed. As I turned towards home, I flashed my headlights on and off twice. They were watching, and I wanted Them confused. I wanted Them to wonder who I was signalling to, to throw Them off my trail.

I drove home. The cop car was gone from our street, the house was quiet.

TEN

My cousin Lesley had been hanging around occasionally for the last couple of months. She was new to Brisbane, having grown up in Clermont, a little mining town in a region that's almost desert. Young people like to escape Clermont for Brisbane if they get the chance, which must be like moving to a different planet. Lesley and I had gone out a few times to the rave clubs that she was getting into. Friday morning she called and said we should do something that night. She'd be over in an hour or so, she said.

While I waited for her to arrive, I went through a box of old magazines that my brother Justin had left at our place. In an old porn magazine, I discovered the pin-up girl was named Lesley. I panicked. Someone was going to hurt her before she arrived. I paced around the house, terrified for her. I recalled something I heard in the lectures about family members of dissidents coming under threat. She'd be attacked. She'd never make it here.

There was nothing I could do. The relief when she made it there safely was enormous. 'Sorry about the mess,' I said, gesturing at the clothes and debris littered all over the place.

'It's OK, you don't have to explain it to me,' she said, smiling.

I gave no indications of being ready to leave.

'Are you going to wear that out tonight?' she prompted. 'Do you want to get some spare clothes?'

At last! She was taking me to a better, safer place, away from the intricate twisted web of enemies and oppression surrounding our house. I was leaving, and it felt permanent. She had come to save me. I grabbed a bag and chucked in some shirts and pants. Lesley lived on the south side, close to the city. As we drove south it was like a weight being lifted off me. The area was more built up, less suburban — for some reason I'd begun to associate suburbia with police-statedom. I seemed to be seeing all this for the first time: the north side was fascist territory. The revolution's borders were somewhere right across the north and south of Brisbane; now we were passing into allied territory. But there was danger here, too, enemies and spies.

I didn't speak much as we drove, instead taking in the surroundings, mapping out the political landscape and enjoying the invigorating sense of freedom, something you could almost taste on the air you breathed. On the car radio was a Fatboy Slim song, which was, naturally, directed at me. It was saying that the time to become aware of revolution, clear as day, around us. Right about now, they were saying. Become aware of the revolution, because it's happening right about now …

When we got to Lesley's place, a small apartment, I sat on the living-room floor, not saying a word — there was so much to take in and process. Lesley told me about an upcoming music festival that staged acts from all genres. She wanted me to perform there. I'd forgotten about my destiny as a musical messiah in the fascist north, but here it could happen. It was a joyous feeling.

Lesley must have run out of ways to make conversation with her silent cousin. She said she had today's newspaper if I wanted to read it.

She was asking me to look through it and spot the articles which were fabrications or cover-ups by the fascist north. I spread out the newspaper on the floor and leaned over it, pawing the pages like an animal. My hands traced over the articles using psychic power to pick which ones were suspect. I didn't read the words, my eyes ran over the text, uncomprehending. I pointed at a few to Lesley, said little or nothing — there was no point, she knew what I was doing. Lesley watched.

A while before Doug, the actor, had shown me a book about animal totems. The animal you feel the most affinity with can represent certain personality traits that you have. At the time I'd realised that the dog was my totem. What made that idea pop into my head at that moment I'm unsure, but as I sat on Lesley's floor pawing over the newspaper, the notion stirred in my imagination and seemed to become real — this was, after all, some kind of spiritual awakening. I was a dog, reverting or elevating closer to that state, running on instinct and heightened senses.

Afternoon came. Lesley had the night planned. She wanted Paul to come along, and a few other mutual friends. We called Paul at work. He didn't want to come at first, he had other things on. I tried to persuade him, because the night out in Brisbane was more than it seemed. Something massive was going to happen. Anyone who was not in the south when the big event occurred would be in serious danger. We had to get everyone we knew across the border. Maybe China was going to drop bombs on the north side, then invade and turn the place into a Communist state. The revolution had been moving north slowly up until now, but things were about to get drastic. Anyone with luxurious possessions would be targeted and shown no mercy.

I mentioned to Lesley that she might want to hide her stereo. She asked me why. I shrugged. Maybe she'd already dealt with people of the upcoming invasion, maybe she and they had an understanding. She was perhaps allowed a few trinkets like this, in exchange for her help. I admired the way she had a mirror placed facing the back door; it was a very clever magical security device to repel attackers.

I called Paul again, almost pleading with him to join us that night. I was worried; he might die if he was left on the north side. Eventually he called back and said he'd come.

'Where are we going to meet?' I asked him.

'We're just going to wander around and look for people we know,' he said. *We're going to form a clan of like-minded people. If we all band together, we'll survive, even flourish.* Paul was in the know after all, part of something hidden, but an ally. How had he come across all the secret plans? How did he know about the coming disaster, and the part our group would play? I pictured an urban life as a wanderer in a doomed postwar city. We'd travel in gangs, scavenging what food we could. We'd need pack mentality to survive. From now on it would be each clan on its own.

I watched some television while Lesley got ready for the big night. Unknown to me, she called my mother from her bedroom and told her she was very worried about me. Something was wrong, she said, but she didn't know what. Mum asked her if she was sure. I'd seemed fine last time she'd seen me, Mum said.

The Channel Nine news was on. It was the weather report. I stared into the presenter's eyes. He stared back into mine. I knew he could see me; his smile was taunting. I stared back with an evil, hungry grin. I stood up and approached the television, towering over it. The presenter stumbled over his words.

'… psychotic … er, *cyclonic* winds …'

I did a kind of war dance. Bent knees, stalking steps, martial-arts hand gestures, an open challenge. They could see every move — I knew it, they knew it. Here we were, naked before each other at last. The ads came on. The last one was an ad for the movie showing that night, *Godzilla*. On the screen a giant stomping foot pounded down onto the road, crushing pavement. 'TONIGHT!' the voiceover said.

Godzilla? It was all real, I knew it. A nuke was being dropped on the south side tonight. The fascists were striking back. That ad was a message from them, warning anti-revolutionaries to head north, right away. *Leave, and hurry!* it was saying. *There's no time. We are going to blast the south side and wipe out the revolution in one hit.* I got shivers down my spine in waves, fascinated by the revelation, by the fact I could perceive it. America was evacuating the south and about to bomb it.

Lesley came into the lounge room and asked if I was ready to go. I said I was, bracing myself for a tough journey. She asked if I was going to put some shoes on. I hadn't brought any — it hadn't even occurred to me. I didn't know what to do. Lesley thought for a moment, then said we'd better go back to my place and get them. I asked her if she was sure I'd need them. She said that yeah, I probably would. We got back in the car and headed north. The rush-hour traffic confirmed what I knew: people were fleeing the city in droves.

A storm was brewing. The clouds were an oppressive grey-black. Thunder began booming from the west. As we drove north rain lashed down hard over the windscreen, the wipers hardly keeping up. I felt tired suddenly. I closed my eyes and tried to sleep. Lesley was saying comforting words. Again I felt myself reverting to the state of my animal totem. Lesley's words lost all meaning. Her voice was soothing and comforting, but I heard no words. Like a dog I heard her tones and her pitch, that was all: '… it's all right, bla da su in ma deah, foh meh di ah …'

We got out of the city and back on the main road to the northern suburbs. The rain was absolutely bucketing down. Traffic was backed up, roads already waterlogged. Many utes and trucks passed us packed to the brim with possessions. People were stocking up with supplies and heading to the mountains to avoid the holocaust. They'd seen the warning on the news. We were caught in a big traffic jam. Lesley said she wished I'd brought my shoes with me.

Then her car broke down. Someone with a remote control somewhere sent a signal to her car, deliberately stranding us so we couldn't escape the coming danger. On her mobile phone she tried calling the RACQ but couldn't get through.

Eventually some police drove past and saw us. Terror as they pulled over. They got out and offered us some help. My eyes were fixed on the guns in their holsters. They were about to execute us, as soon as there weren't any witnesses to see it. Traffic was moving freely now — it wouldn't be long.

The police were friendly and polite. They stood at either side of the bonnet and pushed the car onto the traffic island. They asked Lesley if she knew anyone who could come and pick us up. She said she did. The cops left us there to wait for the real executioner; they, it seemed, had just put us in position.

Standing on the traffic island in the rain as the cars sped past, splashing water up onto it. This was the end. The rain tasted sweet. It was chemicals I was tasting — America was flying overhead, poisoning the water in the sky, making it rain down in a mist onto everything below. Rather than lose an ally to Communism, they were going to kill everyone here.

Some way in the distance, across the lanes of the drenched road, there was another car broken down. A tow truck was flashing its yellow lights. Lesley pointed at the yellow lights and sadly told me they indicated I'd alerted the authorities of the revolution. My war dance before the TV had been reckless, irresponsible, a petty little battle to prove my power over the television. I should have played things more carefully. My heart sank. I had killed the revolution myself, let everyone down. I'd really been working for the enemy this entire time. The yellow lights were a warning signal, alerting the fascists. No bomb was coming, but I'd betrayed everyone.

Cars were now becoming more sparse, the rain still steady but falling lighter now. Lesley kept trying to call people on her mobile, getting worried as it ran out of power. Soon a car would slow down, someone would wind down a window and gun me down, here by the road. 'Don't worry, Will,' Lesley said, seeing the way I wheeled about on the spot, facing every car that passed; I wanted to see it coming.

Be brave, she was saying. It was inevitable, I was going to die, I may as well accept it and take it with dignity. But I couldn't help being afraid, nor feeling slightly betrayed that she'd accept my death so easily.

At last Lesley got through to one of her friends. She'd meet us at the BP station a kilometre or two up the road. Lesley walked in front. I was barefoot, the ground muddy and soft. We were passing through enemy territory. I still feared the cars that passed.

We found the service station, where a lot of people had pulled in to wait for the water to drain away from the flooded road ahead. A hundred metres north a small creek had overflowed.

Lesley spotted her friend Amy's car. Another Clermont refugee, Amy seemed like a military commander, the way she marched around giving instructions. How high did her authority reach? Lesley went and conferred with her as they puzzled out what to do with her broken-down car.

I stood on my own by the footpath. A crowd of people stood near the doors of the servo. A uniformed policeman in the crowd caught my eye — he seemed to nod in my direction. All of them seemed to be watching me. Of course they were. I was again the centre of the universe. I felt awkward, but something had to be done, a signal sent. Slowly I began pacing back and forth, rotating my palms in some kung-fu moves I'd been learning as part of my health kick. My hands cupped the air, waving in front of me slowly and gracefully. I wasn't sure what I was trying to communicate; it was all impulse, but I was certain it meant *something*.

A couple of dozen people stood nearby, peering with curiosity at the guy with the septum piercing dancing slowly out in the rain rather than wait under shelter with everyone else.

Someone got me into Amy's car. We went back to her townhouse in Aspley, not far from the servo, where she lived with her fiancé, John. I couldn't decide if these two were on our side or not; Amy probably was, but John was an alien spy. Amy presumably had him as a servant or pet; a person with her authority wouldn't allow a spy to live undetected in her home. I got the sense that though he'd come trying to act as a subversive agent, he would end up learning Amy's lessons by accident during his stay; she was going to convert him.

While Amy parked the car, Lesley and I waited by the

front door. By the window a small grey cat pawed the glass. I traced my finger over the glass as the cat playfully moved its head, following my finger. Lesley watched me with a concerned look on her face. She told me that the cat was actually robotic, a synthetic UFO spy. Alarmed, I withdrew my hand from the glass and watched the cat suspiciously.

We went upstairs. The others sat at the table and played cards. I lay on the couch. I needed sleep. The cat jumped up on the couch a few times. It was monitoring me, recording data about me, cameras in its eyes recording everything. It had been sent to Earth to study the human being, our mannerisms and thought processes. I let it stay near me but didn't touch it. The others went to bed.

The house was dark and quiet. I had no inclination to reflect on the momentous goings-on, including what had seemed like a near-death experience by the roadside; it had all been so tiring. Yet I couldn't sleep, not with a television in the room, with its hateful camera inside. The TV may as well have been a huge conscious eye, blinking as it stared at me.

I tiptoed around the house, then took a book I'd brought with me from my bag, *Wiccan Mysteries*. As with the newspaper at Lesley's place, I couldn't comprehend the words — the letters were jumbled symbols, saying nothing. I let my eyes skim over the pages, thinking the words would resonate deep in my subconscious, conveying what had to be important instructions.

There was a stuffed toy panda sitting on the floor. I picked it up and examined it. There were cameras placed in its eyes. I held the doll for a minute, thinking, then put the doll face-first before the television. It was a statement, a message for Them: *You watch us, but we watch you.*

The sun came up. I hadn't slept at all.

The intensity of the night's storms would be a common topic of conversation in the following days, particularly the damage done to several car yards, which ran into the hundreds of thousands. It would soon become clear that *I* had caused the storm. *I* had unleashed all that power. When people mentioned it, though there was a touch of awe in their voices, they seemed to do so with an element of warning: *You'd better not do that again.* It worried me. How had I done it the first time? How could I stop myself from doing it again?

We drove back to Lesley's car, still parked on the traffic island. She had the RACQ coming. When they arrived I felt anxious, didn't trust the mechanic, but Lesley seemed reasonably relaxed so I offered no protest. She left with Amy, and John took me home.

STRANGE PLACES

I was confused and disappointed as I got in the car; wasn't I to be taken away from that place for good? Hadn't there been world-changing events overnight? Why did everything look so much like it had before?

We were heading deeper into enemy territory as we went further north. The sky was clear, no storms. Things seemed just that little bit brighter. It was time to consolidate, plan our next moves in the war.

When I arrived home a friend of ours, Charles, was asleep on the couch. He had a few days' worth of facial hair. I wondered if he was a werewolf. I felt a moment of intense and complete respect for him: he had slept in the lounge room *in front of the television*. It showed a courage and nerve I wished I'd possessed the night before: *To hell with the camera, let 'em watch me,* he seemed to be saying.

I went to my room and dozed for an hour or so, though with my brain in overdrive it wasn't easy, no matter how badly I needed sleep. I was alone in the house again when I got up. I sat out the front, shirtless, staring at the row of houses across from us. I saw it clearer than ever: I was sitting on the borderline of the revolution. It stretched further north than I had realised. The road out front *was the very boundary*. Across the street was fascist country.

Less than a kilometre away from our place was the Brothers Holy Spirit football club, where I'd played league as a child. From our front yard it was possible to see one of the light towers, many powerful lights atop a tall pole with a rectangular head. Suddenly I recognised it as a massive weapon. It was facing south, pouring radiation on us.

I had conjured the storm — there had to be a way I could use those immense powers again. I sat cross-legged and closed my eyes. Again shivers surged up and down my spine while I murmured inarticulate sounds. When I opened my eyes I saw something amazing. The lights had changed direction. They now pointed north.

In the afternoon Robert came home with his girlfriend, Kelly. Instinct told me to trust Kelly, she had the air of someone who would protect and guide. She struck me as a witch of a different school from Dawn; white magic, perhaps.

Robert sat down. We talked about last night's storm. 'It was quite a big one,' he said. He removed his glasses, his eyes squinting as they adjusted to their nakedness. There was something so unutterably threatening in his squinting face that I backed away in terror. He was an alien, a cyborg, a robot. He'd been monitoring me this whole time after all, and by creating the storm I'd pushed him too far.

I backed out of the room, down the hall and into my bedroom, where I tried to recover from the shock, regain some composure. That he'd been here the whole time and

STRANGE PLACES

I'd never noticed, that was what scared me ... He knew *everything*. I waited in my room, hoping he'd leave. I listened to the quiet conversation from the next room. The little snatches I heard confirmed everything. Thank God Kelly was here to keep watch on him, influence him. She wouldn't let him hurt me.

I laid low until night. The weather started soaring into storm territory again, the clouds darkening in all directions. I could not stay in the house with the cyborg. I had to go to Paul's place. I packed some notebooks of lyrics into my bag and phoned Paul, but he wasn't home. I asked my protector, Kelly, if I could get a lift there. She said sure, but she'd have to borrow a car, since Robert had gone out on some errand.

I asked Trent if we could use his car. I made gesticulations, believing I was casting a spell on him so he'd let us. He frowned at my waving arms and said sure. Kelly asked me if Trent was an automatic or manual. She meant was he the type who needed magical attention or the type who was simply agreeable without such fanfare. I said he was an automatic. By coincidence, so was his car.

ELEVEN

As we head south to Carseldine the sky looks furious, frantic. Kelly asks me if I have a girlfriend at the moment, looking to set me up with a friend of hers. I laugh and say no; funnily enough this question is exactly as it seems; there are no hidden meanings.

We get to my brother's place in Carseldine as the storm is about to break. Thunder sounds distantly, the first fat drops of rain fall. I get out of the car and wave goodbye to Kelly. I fear for her safety — there will be forces intent on harming her since she has helped me. This storm is not fucking about, it means business, and it isn't my doing this time. But she seems so holy, like a guardian spirit. She brought me here safely, closer to the centre of the storm, closer to the city — that could not have been done without some kind of power. It is best, I decide, that she leave before the situation, the turmoil, gets worse and overcomes her.

STRANGE PLACES

The house in Carseldine is a one-storey brick place. There is a train line just over the back fence, only metres away. Paul and his girlfriend rent the place with a pagan couple, Warren and Kaya. They are spiritual beings, which is good, because if ever I needed spiritual guidance it is now, during war.

Warren and Kaya have a baby daughter. As I approach the front door I hear her loud crying from inside. I can hear their voices in tandem trying to calm her. They sound a little frantic. The baby must fear the storm and the cataclysm, that is what has upset her. It is a bad time to intrude, so I hang around out the front for a while, waiting for the crying to stop. I know better than to upset a ritual.

Some time passes and I knock sheepishly at the door. Eventually it opens and Warren is standing there, tall and thin, dressed in black. His light beard, wild eyes and bushy eyebrows light up in surprise. 'Hey there, man, didn't know you were here.'

I mutter something about the storm and he gestures to come in. The baby has stopped crying. My brother is not home yet, is still at work in town, as is his girlfriend. I drop my bag in a corner of the living room and awkwardly take a seat at the kitchen table. As I look around I see a shelf full of books on Celtic history and witchcraft. On the table there's a bong and a small bowl of cannabis. Inside the house it's quiet and relaxing as the rain drums on the roof. It feels like sanctuary.

Warren and Kaya are talking to me, friendly, polite. But I have no idea what the hell is going on, nor what they're really saying. Everything I say is clouded and vague, but Warren seems to understand. I ask about the books around us, and my gaze fixes on one that has a picture of a marijuana leaf that is blended into the green face of a bearded man. I look around but my eyes keep returning to this book. Something about it is hypnotic. 'Warren,' I say, feeling boisterous suddenly, 'can I have a cone?' I am confident, obeying the strange book's signal.

'If you want to, man, sure.'

The weed is already chopped, mixed with tobacco. I pack a small amount carefully into the cone. I light it up, suck back the smoke, and the harsh attack on my lungs brings tears to my eyes as I cough. It's strong.

'Can I have some more?' I croak.

'Go ahead.'

I put another small amount in the cone, and inhale. It hits fast. I sit there numb, reeling from the chemicals mingling in my brain, all the more powerful for their long absence. My eyes return to the book, the one with the marijuana-leaf face. I see layers in the picture, astonishing depth, as I stare into the aged eyes. I stare and stare, suddenly unable to speak, falling into the picture of the face like it's a star, the face of some Earth-god.

In the background I can hear Warren and Kaya talking. The sounds don't seem to be English anymore, but a kind of secret language, animal noises again, and laughter. It's sometimes soothing, sometimes frightening. I sense they are perusing my thoughts, going through them like the pages of a magazine, reading me. They're reading my mind, chuckling at some parts, making concerned noises at others. Still staring at the face on the book, I *show* them my thoughts. My mind drifts, and I think of the tyre dealer in Strathpine called Dog Tyred, how the name is a ploy to sedate people passing by and lower their resistance to a police state. I show them the signals from the television, what the ads *mean*. I want them to see what it all means. I show them everything.

They pace around the room. Each thought I present is met with either a burst of laughter, or a concerned groan, or an inquisitive noise. I am not scared. These are my spiritual authorities here. Warren is my mentor. My master. All-knowing. Wise. I am his apprentice, and he will teach me.

I don't know how my trance is broken, but I am feeling ill when I break free. I look around gingerly. Warren suggests heading outside for a smoke. I somehow stand upright, make it to a chair outside the back door. Warren follows me. The rain is pattering steadily. I light a cigarette, the first I've smoked in a few months. Next to me Warren is saying something about a role-playing game called Werewolf: the Masquerade. I cannot hear him properly, I am too far gone. I am staring at the trees in the backyard ... and holy shit, look at them. They're like shapes you see in clouds, only more real. They are *alive*. The magnitude of this blows my mind. The shapes, shapes of animals in the trees, they're so vivid.

I sit back in my chair, head spinning as I look above me at the dark outlines. There is one that looks like a wolf with a baby on its back. That's me. I am the wolf. The baby is Warren's baby. I am its guardian. I am the dog. I am clearing a path for her, the child ... that is what this fight is all about. I am a servant, a protector.

The other shapes ... there is a panda. It is the largest of them all, overlooking the rest with something like menace. It is ... China. China is coming, China is watching us all. The weight of this, the significance, falls on me heavily. China is here, awake and colossal. The revolution has begun, slowly and surreptitiously, about to become a stampede. The area around us now is a war zone, a silent war. The forces that reside here are cut off from the forces of the West. The new age, China, here, encompassing ... my God.

Other shapes in the trees: the bird, perched facing opposite the dog-steed. It is watching, silently, a guardian. It is woman. It is fighting in the revolution from a different front. Its head is pointed my way, and it seems to have a finger raised to its mouth in a *hush* gesture. I must be silent. The fight is silent; I understand, Tree-Goddess.

The other shapes, all so *alive*, so real. I am reeling with these revelations. I don't notice that gradually I am leaning forward, my head almost between my knees ...

Werewolf. Warren is talking about werewolves.

It is coming. I am becoming a werewolf. I can feel my teeth lengthening, my jaw jutting out, the pain wracking me. My eyes are shut as I await the transformation. My body wrenches, lunges forward from within. This is my initiation. I am becoming a wolf. The thought frightens me, but I accept. I mouth the words: 'I accept, I accept, I accept.'

For an age I sit there as the pain and straining have their way with my body. Any moment I will run wild, senses keen as blades, and I will hunt.

'Are you all right, man?' Warren's voice interrupts, cutting through background sounds. It's almost a shock to hear comprehensible language. My eyes open and I'm staring at my shoes, body bent forward in a foetal position. I turn around and look up at him, standing by the doorway.

'You OK, man? You wanna come in and watch a movie? We're gonna watch a movie — why don't you come inside?'

I pull myself upright with effort. My steps are clumsy and tentative as I go inside.

'Can you shut the door, man?'

I've left it open, and feel a pang of shame. Then it becomes colossal guilt. Mosquitoes may have gotten in — they may harm the baby. She might get sick and die. I have broken a rule, like a bad guard dog. *Bad dog.* I slide the insect screen shut, and stagger to the lounge room. I lie down on the couch in front of the television, Warren and Kaya sitting on the couch to the left. Warren puts on a movie. I can't watch it in this state. I close my eyes and listen to the dialogue.

The movie, I soon discover, is made by someone from deep within the system. To my horror, it is a satire not just of my resistance, but the resistance of everyone who fights the powers that govern us. The movie is called *Scary Movie*. Every burst of laughter from Warren and Kaya is mocking damnation to me. The movie clearly parallels every thought I have recently had — even my mind's response to one line of the movie is instantly mocked by the next line of dialogue. I lie there silently, humiliated, eyes closed, and drift into restless sleep.

I remember vaguely being awoken at some point by visitors. They look like Kaya's parents. These people are vampires, I realise groggily, perhaps come to feed from me. They may bite me, they may not; it doesn't matter much. I pretend that I am still asleep on the couch as they talk quietly to Warren and Kaya, and soon enough sleep comes again. The visitors leave.

Of what came next, I am not sure how much is dream, or hallucination, or reality.

Outside the moon is full. I am out there by the back door, guarding. I am part of the clan now, a new member. Warren's clan. We are either wolves, or we are *like* wolves — it is not yet clear which. I am outside because I haven't earned the right to sit inside. I haven't yet hunted and brought the clan food. I left the door open. I am sitting out here as punishment. But I will guard the clan with all my heart, with my life; part of me yearns for the chance to fight and prove it.

The world is at war. Soon, there will be no laws. It will be each clan for themselves, all scavenging what's left when the war destroys everything. Clans are forming all over in preparation. There are the inner-city clans, who feed mercilessly on anyone who crosses into their domain. There are the bush clans, who live from the land and survive in the wild, setting traps for those who accidentally blunder into their territory. In the suburbs there are families who band together, neighbours who find refuge with each other. These are the weakest, the most vulnerable, and so are often the prey of the others. There are police, a brutal clan from which the likes of us hide. The biker clans, fearsome rangers, roamers. There are the rich, the worst of all. These use all the others and crush opponents, set the rules of the game, change them as it suits.

All this conflict is brewing, a tension which can almost be seen in the air. Survival will be a battle between all these clans before the backdrop of a new world war, which will destroy social order forever. It is coming like a storm. As I guard the back of the house, all of these realisations come to me, one by one, as neatly and clearly as a puzzle forming from jagged pieces, dropping into place, a huge but vivid new picture of the world.

At some point, I look up and see the moon explode. It has been detonated by America, a nuclear strike. There is no telling why. I actually see it come apart; a white ring of force from the explosion races silently across the sky, growing wider and wider like a giant ripple. That is the signal, it has begun. I rush inside, where Kaya sits on the couch. She is breast-feeding her baby; Warren is pacing, anxious. 'They did it?' he says. Kaya is agitated, trying to contain her temper. 'Yes, they did it.'

They are talking about the destruction of the moon. I lie on the couch and watch them. I realise to my horror I have left the door open *again* ... mosquitoes will attack the baby and make it sick. I feel like a murderer, and rise to close the door, but Warren already has. I struggle for something to say. 'Warren ...'

'What is it, man?'

'Last night ...' My thoughts go to the moon, the open door. 'The baby did it, right?'

'Oh, yeah,' he says, looking at me strangely, the way you'd humour a drunk. 'Yeah, the baby did it.'

I lie on the couch, flustered by these events. It's still dark, though the night seems to have lasted longer than it should. My brother hasn't come home yet. Warren and Kaya talk quietly. I'm mortified, sensing I have done something wrong by my clan.

At some point, while I am drifting between sleep and wakefulness, Warren stands over me in the lounge room. '*Will*,' he says urgently, '*Will*, guard the door! Go!'

My eyes open wide. I look at him, start to rise from the couch, and then I charge. With a burst of energy I leave my body, my spirit bolts out the door, and I pace frantically in the yard, silently challenging anything to come out and try to harm the house or the baby or Warren or Kaya. Master said, 'Guard'. I will guard with my life. Warren has drawn me out of my body, and as I pace back and forth, I am a higher life form, naked spirit.

I wake up and find myself lying on the couch, head clouded. Warren and Kaya have gone to bed. The car pulling into the driveway is presumably what woke me. Car headlights sweep past the window, partly illuminating the dark living room. Paul is home. It's just after 10 pm.

He enters — 'Hey, wassup?' and goes into his bedroom to change out of his work clothes. Groggily I get up, wander around the house, and soon Paul joins me outside. Rain drums lightly on the back patio roof. We light cigarettes. 'You going to play this werewolf game we got coming up?' he says.

'Yeah,' I say. My voice is a croak, my throat not used to the smoke. Words are meaningless. He's speaking in code, but at least I can understand the language and answer in kind. 'But I don't know which clan.'

After more chatter about this, confusion hits. There are too many signals, too many meanings and omens, no definite solid truth for me to use as a reference point. To take a stance in any direction, about any subject at all, seems dangerous. If you asked me if I preferred vanilla or strawberry, I wouldn't have an answer for you; it would seem too risky. After a brief silence I ask, 'Paul, am I doing the right thing?'

He frowns. 'The right thing? What?'

His confusion throws me further adrift. Surely he knows of this strange test I am being put through; surely he sees it all: the coming war, the clan wars. Everyone does. I start to think he's being coy. I try to ask from a different angle. 'I mean, family is important to me …'

He frowns again. 'Well, yeah. It fuckin' should be.'

'So, am I doing the right thing?'

'The right thing? What? What do you mean?'

After a moment I understand what he's saying. There *is* no right thing. There is only what is right for the clan, only survival.

We go inside, into the living room. Paul packs some pot into the bong and starts smoking. I consider warning him about the camera in his television. They are watching him perform an illegal act. He is a marked man, it's recorded on camera. But he appears to know more than I do about how it all works, so I say nothing. 'You wanna watch the Broncos game? I taped it.'

I don't object. He says he can't stand the TV commentary. He puts on a CD, mutes the television, sticks in the tape, and the game starts. A horrific scene unfolds. The lyrics to the song on his stereo form a dreadful connection to the body language of the footballers on the screen. It is all threat. A player smiles at the camera after scoring a try, pointing a finger skyward — *You are dead, matey*. The band is Ween, the song 'Piss Up a Rope', a country/western parody.

Paul played this music for a reason. He is worldly, knows the ins and outs of the system. At his job, he is among it. I have broken a serious law. I am now going to pay.

I opt to challenge this threat. I make jokes about the football game. I mock the players on screen. Paul's responses, though I can't recall the words, mean: *Don't say that, you are making it worse. They're going to get you. They're coming for you. It can't be avoided now.*

The Brisbane Broncos football team are on their way here to cut my testicles off and/or kill me. I ask Paul in oblique ways how I can stave off this oncoming attack. I get no clues because he is going to bed soon. Been a long day. He says I am to face it myself, it is not his problem.

He leaves me on the couch with this familiar sinking feeling. I am hunted again. I am scared again. I'm sick of feeling like this. I turn off all lights in the room and sit on the floor out of view of the camera (television). I sit by the window in the dark, quiet house, streetlights dimly outlining the window. Every now and then a car passes, and I am sure this is the one. A car will pull into the driveway, doors will open and a bunch of huge men will jump out, shouting my name, kicking down the door, dragging me outside, pulling my legs apart and slicing my dick off with knives. With each set of headlights that flashes by this certainty builds, and I sit in the dark, alone, terrified.

I remember the clan. My attackers must *not* come inside the house. I must face them on my own; this is my fight, this is a sentence for some crime. I know too much. But if harm comes to me I will not let it come to my clan. I have to face the threat outside, on my own.

I rise to my feet, feeling a surge of adrenaline, knowing this is the last hour — at most — of my life. I stalk through the house silently, trying to invoke the wolf in myself, the wolf that ran free of my body earlier. The wolf can fight them ... maybe. My feet are balanced, the muscles in my legs feel hard as I prowl to the kitchen. There I slide two small kitchen knives out of the rack and hold them expertly, one in each hand. I examine my weapons, I kiss them. My heart is racing like never before. The fight for my life approaches. I will not go down without fighting back.

Every move I make now is deliberate, stealthy. My powers are awakening. I slide the door open, step outside. Tessa, Paul's dog, looks at me curiously. I wave her away, tell her to hush. She does. I am wolf, I can command my kindred.

The moon is full above me ... this does not register. Now I survive, not think. I walk out into the yard; a strut, a defiant saunter. They can see me, I am sure of that. They have come here silently, and surround the house now. I feel them.

In the middle of the yard, surrounded, vulnerability spurs me into a heightened state. I hold the blades clear for them to see. I hear a noise in the bushes behind me. I turn around, fast as a cat, and point my blade. Over my shoulder, another noise. I turn to face it, knife raised. My body issues challenges. I begin something of a dance, a silent war cry. Fear and adrenaline fuel my movements, but they are controlled, every one bearing meaning. I stomp, spinning around in a circle, knives whistling in the air. My movements increase in speed, sometimes a graceful dance, like a martial artist, sometimes jagged, casually brutal.

Every time I hear a noise in a bush, or from over the back fence, I wheel about, stop, face it, smile at it. *Oh no you don't, I see you.* I wave my knives at it, and wait for the next.

These are malevolent spirits around me, I realise. Ghost forms. This may be a test set by my clan, testing my worth as a fighter. Maybe they will kill me and I will be reborn as a vampire. Live or die, I must earn their respect.

Soon I am spinning around in a circle, forming a mental picture of a circle around me, drawn out with my blades. Inside this circle, no harm can come to me. It is a spell I have cast, a circle of protection. I grin at the spirits around me, and step out of the circle to expose myself. *Come and get me.*

The dance increases in energy. In the yard Tessa is running around madly in a wide circle, not barking, but bolting fast around and around the yard. I slap the flats of the knife blades against my skin, my wrists. I make scratches in time with the rhythm, trying to draw blood. To the shadows around me I display this; I draw the metal across my wrists, showing them I have no fear of pain or blood. A train passes, noise like thunder, yellow-lit windows visible as they go by. I make scissor-like motions towards the train with my knives in one hand. Then I make the same motion above my crotch. Another spell. It means: *You take mine, I take yours. I take your* technology. My gestures feel ancient, magical.

Blood starts to trickle. My cuts become deeper and sting. A plane flies overhead, and I raise my wrists above my head, and taste myself. The plane is a vampire in disguise; I am a vampire too.

I dig the blades into the ground and smear dirt on my wounds, rubbing it up the thin cuts on my wrists. I rub some on my face, feeling primal, tribal. I take off my shirt, hide the blades under it, and incorporate this into the ritual.

Gradually, I tire. My tiredness makes me vulnerable and clumsy. The attack has not come yet; why must they wait for me to be too tired? Why can't they fight me when I am at my peak? It isn't fair. I wander back into the house. I turn around in a circle, blades pointed downwards, casting my spell again. *No harm can come to me from within here*, I try to incant. But my powers feel weak, and the spell does not take hold inside. Instinct tells me to leave the house.

I am exhausted as I step back outside. My arms are hurting from the dirt I rubbed into the cuts. Drizzle has begun to fall. I let it douse my heated skin, steam coming off it. My walk isn't stealthy or calculated anymore. It's now slumped and exhausted. I head to the side of the house and lean against it. I sit there and wait for the car to pull up, and for my attackers to come. I still have my knives ready for when they do, but I have lost my energy.

Thoughts drift. The revolution is nothing glorious. It is a dirty war of survival. I have offended spiritual forces beyond my reckoning. I am succumbing to defeat. My mind replays some old song lyrics: *So should they find me, back to the wall / What's left inside me, will come to call / And as the blood spills, as the life drains / All who bear witness, will know my name.*

It is prophecy. I chant the last line, its meaning dawning on me gradually. It is a final call to arms, one last challenge. 'All who bear witness, will know my name.' The words come out in a whisper. I repeat them, over and over. 'All who bear witness, *Will, know my name.*' My name, Will, is the struggle. Witness my suffering, and know the secrets. This is what it means.

'*All who bear* — witness Will — *know my name.*' All who bear … children. Women. All women will see. They have the power of the moon. They will know my name. The mothers. Their power is greater than all.

All who bear … burden. Your struggle is mine. I am the catalyst of your fight. Your Messiah. Witness my death, know my name.

'All who bear witness, *will know* my name.' Aha, this time it is a warning. To those who perpetuate this evil, beware; the rest *will know*. They will see. Your fall will follow mine.

I chant until the words lose all meaning, the syllables merge into a flowing inarticulate murmur, an incantation, as I flick away the incessant, merciless mosquitoes with my knives.

Rain comes down in a slow, steady mist. I sit cross-legged on the grass, back to the brick wall, knives in each hand. Mosquitoes swarm around me, biting my shins and calves. I let them. These bites are punishment. Each one sucks my blood until the pain gets too much, and then I whimper and slap them. Someone is punishing me, and I deserve it. The mosquitoes are relentless, and with each bite I find myself saying the words 'I'm sorry.' Sorry for being weak, when I should have been strong. Sorry for being the dog that I am. I wrap my arms around my knees, let them bite me, whimper, slap them away. I do this for hours until the first light of day begins to appear.

The spirits start to talk to me. Not in the form of voices, just in thoughts.

What are you doing here?

I am a guardian, I tell them.

You're weak. Why are you weak?

I am a dog, I tell them. I am not a leader; I obey.

Good, well you go into the shed, and you die, dog.

I don't protest. I nod solemnly, and walk over to the garden shed. The spirits' words hurt me, they are so unforgiving. Tessa the dog is at my heels, looking at me inquisitively as I open the shed door and go inside. It is musty, dark and cramped in here. Garden tools lie scattered, and there is camping equipment. I unroll a foam mattress, and I sit in there for a while, Tessa keeping me company.

It's time to die. I hold the knife to my wrist, and try to cut myself. The skin won't break. I don't understand it. My arm, is it bionic? Is my skin made of something stronger? I dig around in the scratches I have already made. The blood won't come.

I feel something sting my foot; a redback spider has bitten me. The shed's floor is brick, the spiders nest down in the cracks between them. I barely notice the bite. I am too busy processing that death won't come to me today. I'm not relieved by this, just confused. I look around the shed. Camping equipment … Maybe I have to head for the bush, live off the land. I make vague lists of what I will need to survive in the wild. Visions of life as a wanderer come to me; roaming the streets, the bush, visiting houses of friends from time to time for shelter in rough weather. It is an intriguing prospect.

I notice an old folder lying on the floor, and I open it. It contains drawings from an old art class, which are plans to redesign reality. The implications are serious ... I have discovered another major revelation, secrets of global importance. I hope that I haven't hindered these plans in any way by discovering the drawings — I have brought other grand plans undone with my mistakes already.

I see why these drawings are stored in the shed, and not the camera-infested house. In the shed infrared beams from satellites will be unable to penetrate. Yet I fear for the safety of these secrets. No doubt the people watching me have seen me in here, and will soon discover these drawings. I visualise the police cars which will arrive at any moment, taking the secret drawings away, me with them. It is time to leave the shed.

I pick up the mattress, which I will need when living in the wilderness. Tessa's nose is covered in spider webs from sniffing around in the shed's dusty corners. The sun is up now, but no police have arrived yet. As I walk towards the house the pain in my foot from the spider bite starts to flare up. The pain is intense, like having a lit cigarette pressed there.

Kaya opens the front door to answer my knock. I ask her if I can sleep in the garage next to the house. She looks concerned. I realise she is concerned because I have been in the shed, and discovered the plans to redesign reality. She nods though, and agrees I can sleep in the garage.

STRANGE PLACES

I wander through the house, starting to feel dizzy from the spider bite and from physical exhaustion. I roll the mattress out on the concrete floor of the garage, though it's far too small for me, and say goodnight to Kaya. I will have to leave when I wake, leave for the bush. I sleep.

TWELVE

After about four hours of blackness I wake up in the garage to the smells of dust and my own sweat. As I rise from the concrete floor I can hear the muffled voices of the household ... Paul, Warren, Kaya, and Paul's girlfriend. Inside the house I am greeted with casual *good mornings*. Paul offers coffee, I decline. My mind feels clouded, sedate, a mild hangover from yesterday's pot.

I sit outside and smoke a cigarette with Paul. After some small talk about the werewolf game I ask if I can rest in his bed for a while. He doesn't mind, and I lie there waiting for more sleep. The soft sheets feel heavenly on my insect-bitten legs.

Out the window I can see the backyard, and suddenly I remember the night before. I wonder if they saw my dance with the knives, and what they thought. Did they approve of my performance? No harm came to the household, to the clan, after all. I fended off the attack, the onslaught … for now. Yet part of me feels it was never the clan's fight, it was my own. I sleep again.

When I wake, I hear Paul talking to my parents. I don't know what they are doing here, yet the sight of my mother reassures me. A familiar sight, a trusted sight. I walk outside to the back patio where she, Paul, Warren and Kaya are in conversation. Everyone goes quiet for a moment as I take a seat. Mum smiles at me, asks me how I am.

I sit and smoke, and ask what's going on.

'Paul called me, love,' Mum says. 'He was concerned about you. How do you feel?'

I answer that I don't know. 'Is Dad here?'

'He's gone to get us some lunch — fish and chips.'

I sit quietly with my clan around me. What part my mother plays in all this I am unsure, but I don't question why she is here. I feel some sort of calmness, some reassurance from the conversation going on around me. Mum notices the army of red welts on my legs from the mosquito bites. She says there will be some well-fed mosquitoes flying home this morning. My legs are itching badly. I sit, relaxed. Mum is here for a *reason*, but I can't guess what it is, or how she fits into all these secret wars. It just seems safe now that she's here.

The reason Mum is here of course is to take me to hospital. This is the deepest state of psychosis I've encountered, far beyond the earlier episode when the television came to life and spoke to me. If I'd been neck-deep then, now I'm caught in a rip and being pulled towards the horizon. There is a chance I'm not coming out of it this time.

Mum tells me she is going to take me to see a doctor. I don't protest, although this news is vaguely frightening; what the hell is a 'doctor'? I rise from my chair, looking for a place to dispose of my cigarette butt. I walk out into the yard. Everyone watches my movements closely, and a sense of purpose blends into the moment. I ceremoniously sink my cigarette into an ant hole, and stand there watching it, performing another ritual, something related to lighting a symbolic fuse to strike the enemies of our clan.

Mum says, 'Honey, do you want to have some lunch or go to the hospital straight away?'

I don't feel like eating, I tell her. She stands, says goodbye to Paul and the others.

'Come on, love,' she says. 'Let's go.'

Panic starts again. I have no idea where we're going, but the word 'hospital' conjures many images. Paul, Warren and Kaya say goodbye, and Paul tells me he'll be in touch. They all seem to know what's going on, though I have no clue; it feels sinister. All I can do is contain the panic and follow my mother out to the car.

Dad has arrived, is standing out the front with a paper parcel of fish and chips in his hand. He says hello. In that moment I realise I have escaped death, for the food he has is poisoned. 'You're leaving now?' he says.

'Yes, you want to follow us?' Mum answers.

Mum asks me which car I want to ride in. I choose hers. I ask repeatedly where we are going, and Mum tells me we're headed for the Prince Charles Hospital. On the drive there my senses begin to awaken again, emerging from the sedated comfort of Paul's back patio. Behind us I see Dad in the other car, and it occurs to me that he is some sort of cyborg, like Robert. There are dozens like him all over the city. His face looks like it's made of metal and plastic.

I stir in my seat. Beside me Mum answers my questions, assuring me that I'll be all right, that I'll be safe. At one point it occurs to me that the storms are coming again, this time in genuinely cataclysmic proportions, that I am one of the few being taken to a safe place — I note that we seem to be driving uphill. A place of high ground, away from the coming floods. I almost see them: waves, mountain-high, sweeping down on us.

We pull into the hospital car park. Dad's car pulls in beside us, and my belief that he is a cyborg is forgotten. Dad's face once again looks like something familiar and safe in this new, unknown place. I walk with my parents to the mental health unit of the Prince Charles Hospital, separate from the main hospital building. Mum goes in to see the receptionist. I wait outside with Dad, smoking cigarettes and trying to interpret my new surroundings. It seems alien, the tall white buildings, concrete passageways, fluorescent lights.

Dad makes conversation. I am both oblivious to its actual meaning and responsive to his lines in my own internal script. I feel like an animal again. I begin to pace around out the front of the mental health building, sometimes crouching and leaping up to touch the roof. The feeling of animalism grows, and I let it govern my movements, my speech. I don't walk … I prowl. I sit with my muscles tense, ready to leap like a tiger. The attitude is a playful one, not aggressive, though it must look strange, even threatening.

Mum comes out the sliding doors and tells me to come in and see the doctor. My parents ask if I want them to accompany me, and I do. In a small room, bare but for some chairs, there is a doctor, a slender thirty-something man, sitting in the corner. He greets us all, and watches me closely. He asks me various personal details: my age, my address, if I have any tattoos, allergies. I stare into his eyes and grin, trying to unsettle him with body language, for he scares me. It is all I can do to stay calm.

The doctor continues his assessment.

'William, do you know why you are here?'

'I am just *here*,' I tell him.

'Do you know the reason you are here? The reason you were brought here?'

I lean forward, and look the doctor in the eye. What I say next seems to bear the weight of the entire world. 'There *is* no reason.'

No reason I was here, no reasoning with me. My mind was its own individual sphere, outside of and alien to the rest of the world. No words or persuasion could change that, or bring me out of this personal universe. I was at the centre, the nucleus, and the only one there, completely alone. All else were stage props and an audience, impersonal and inhuman, sometimes applauding, sometimes howling for blood, but the play was real.

The doctor leaves the room to consult with colleagues, admin staff, and leaves me with my parents. The animal feeling subsides. My parents ask if there's anything I want brought from my place, if I have enough cigarettes, if I want any books or magazines. I don't know. I don't know what's going on, what's about to happen, even though it's explained to me in the plainest English possible.

Dad left the hospital to go and collect some of my things from home. A male nurse, a tall bald man whose smiling face seemed featureless and alien, introduced himself and accompanied my mother and me on a tour of my new home.

The hospital was divided into east and west wings, something my mind seized on immediately, dissecting political implications. It was all one-storey and looked futuristic, space-age. I was shown where I could sit outside and smoke, where I could watch television (no thanks), where the table tennis tables were. The dining area, the recreation rooms, the laundry room, the courtyard. Other patients were mostly in their rooms by now. Those I saw shuffled around in nightgowns, pyjamas and slippers. When they spoke it was in flat voices, nearly monotone, slightly too loud.

My room had a narrow bed, dresser drawers, a closet, private shower and toilet, a window overlooking the courtyard, a desk and chair. It was a homey, cosy-looking place — the perfect cover for something sinister. Like a gas chamber. My bald nurse was a Nazi, and death awaited if I stayed in this trap. There was no way in hell I'd spend the night here.

As a defence, I began thinking that by divine power no harm could come to me. Any person who attempted it would instead fall victim to their own attack; if someone tried to shoot me, the bullet would strike them instead. I was invincible.

I sat with Mum near reception as we waited for Dad to return. He arrived with a box of notebooks and folders and some clothes. In my room they said their goodbyes. They would visit tomorrow, they told me, and bring the rest of my things.

When they were gone I nervously explored the hospital. I went out into the courtyard, sat by the door and smoked, keeping to myself and avoiding the other patients. A young man with a goatee sat beside me and tried to start a conversation. I offered him a cigarette. The slightly amused look in his eye indicated he understood I was off the planet just then. He tried several times to talk to me without getting a coherent response, then paused, pondering a way through the illness's webs. 'I am bipolar,' he said at last.

'I am psychotic,' I replied, attaching my own internal meaning to the word. It was as though we'd exchanged names.

'Psychotic as in kill a lot of people?' he said, smiling.

I smiled at this but didn't answer; maybe he took it to mean 'yes'. There was no more talk until he thanked me for the smoke and went inside.

The bald nurse, the one I was most afraid of, came outside. He was built like a bouncer. Something in me wanted to challenge him, instil respect. I brushed past him, squared up to him, and looked him in the eye. *I am not afraid of you*, my body language said. Rest assured, he was not afraid of me either. Well used to strange behaviour, he smiled placidly and let me pass.

Medication time came. Another large male nurse — there seemed to be quite a few of those around — sat behind a counter in the hallway distributing tablets. He smiled as he handed me two capsules. For a brief moment some visual trick was played: as he emptied his palm into mine, it looked like there were no capsules at all. On second glance I saw the coloured tablets in my palm and looked up at him, startled by his magic trick. Someone in line behind me said something about a wizard. The nurse just smiled and handed me a cup of water. I put the capsules under my tongue, drank the water, walked back to my room and spat out the medication. Medication meant sleep, and sleep meant death.

I sat on my bed for a while, thinking. This place, this

'hospital', was a refuge in a war zone. More than that, it was a POW camp. The war was going on outside the hospital, that infinite fight, left wing versus right wing, clan versus clan, heaven versus hell ... This hospital was a resting place for wounded soldiers of the war, like me. To the south the Communist revolution was gaining ground, and to the north the fascist Fourth Reich stood like a fortress.

I could not stay here. I grabbed my cigarettes and headed back out to the courtyard. There was a gate around the side, unlocked — in a hospital like this, patients usually understand they are safest here, and don't often feel a need to escape. A couple of the other patients sat around in pyjamas, chain-smoking. I tried to look inconspicuous, smoking along with the others. A course of action was forming — nothing conceptually difficult, just walk out the door, but it required the summoning of courage. I walked around the courtyard. An elderly female patient sat slumped and defeated on a white plastic chair. I crouched beside her, feeling like Jesus, and asked her if she was OK. She didn't respond, just stared down at the table in front of her. Somehow, this was a signal: it was time. I nodded to her, said some words of comfort, and then stepped through the gate of the courtyard into a covered walkway.

I walked past hospital buildings that loomed up beside me. Through the windows, snipers waited in position, ready to fire. For a moment the fear was nearly crippling, till I remembered my animal powers; any bullet fired at me would instead strike the gunman.

I found my way to the car park. It was quiet and empty but for a dozen cars spread out across it, lit up by the moon and the hospital's fluorescent lights. No other people were around. Which way was the front gate?

Ahead of me were the back fences of houses on the hospital's perimeter. I headed down a steep embankment towards the fences, preparing to jump over and escape through the yards of the houses. Halfway down the embankment I stopped as headlights flashed behind me. A car pulled up, with two security guards in the front seats.

'What are you doing down there, mate?' one of them said.

I headed back up towards the car, not sure of what to tell them. 'I wanted to see what was down there.'

'What wing are you from?' they asked me. 'East or west?'

I had to use my powers on these men, mentally dominate them. I leaned forward, buoyed by a sudden burst of confidence and power. 'West,' I said, hissing the word.

'What room, mate?'

STRANGE PLACES

'Third.'

That would throw them. West, third … the Western world, the Third Reich; the connections snapped into place. What they were really asking is whose side I was on in the war. In response I had lied and told them I was on their side. They would think I was an ally.

'Slip back for us, would you, mate?' they said.

Slip back into your human form. I nodded, and walked slowly back in the direction from which I'd come. The car moved away, and when it was out of view I about-faced and went down the road, looking for the exit, walking faster. I found a footpath that led out of the hospital and followed it into the night.

My bare feet stepped over bindis and bitumen as I headed up a hilly stretch of road, past houses. The houses looked strange, but somehow seemed not a part of the great war, with their lights on, open doors, and the sounds of music, the smells of cooking; it seemed pagans must live there, people like Warren and Kaya. I walked through a park, below a huge fig tree, bats rustling the leaves above.

At the Gympie Road intersection, I was faced with a problem: I didn't really know where I was going, or which way to turn. Several kilometres to the right was the city, the left led to the north, but I didn't know that — these streets were no longer familiar. I crouched down, closed my eyes, and tried to *sense* which direction I should go. Instinct said left. I followed the road to the end, back out onto the main street.

I passed a construction site where a church was being built. The cross on the sign out front seemed sinister; the war-zone atmosphere grew. I was on the north side now, home of the Fourth Reich, enemy territory. The people inside a laundromat looked through the glass at me as I passed, but didn't seem to see me. I was blending into the night around me, completely invisible, again becoming the wolf I'd been in Paul's backyard.

The cars that passed didn't see me either. I bounded across roads with great speed, hardly pausing to check whether it was safe, certain that if I was struck I could not be hurt. The strength in my legs felt superhuman. Traffic was sparser further north along Gympie Road. When animal instinct dictated, I would sprint across the six-lane road, sensing one side was momentarily safer than the other. Then I would cross back for the same reason.

I came to a service station, the BP Lesley and I had come to the night of the flood, and sat at the footpath out front for a moment's rest. Pedestrians walked past, and I assessed them, judging them to be no threat. Across the road a group of three men walked by, chatting and laughing. Enemies, their style of dress told me. I sprinted across the road, pursuing them, not sure what had to be done when I caught up with them. They saw me and walked faster, turning up a side street, disappeared from view. Victory.

The journey resumed. I still had no destination in mind. I passed Marchant Park, a huge collection of cricket fields, a place where I had played club cricket only a few years before. Now it looked dark and brooding. There were bats in the trees above me. Vampires. The place was infested with vampires. I felt vulnerable. I mustered the strength to combat them. As I walked, every now and then I would turn a circle, casting a ring of protection about myself, the same spell I'd cast during my knife-dance in Paul's backyard. No harm would come to me if I did this vigilantly. But they were following, I could feel it. And I could see the bats overhead, hear them swooping out of the trees.

The path on which I walked deviated from the road, the passing cars further away now. Part of me wanted to run into the midst of the cricket fields and join the vampires, become one of them. They kept following, but did not attack.

After some time I realised I was heading back to Paul's place in Carseldine. I'd walked about ten kilometres along the road, my bare feet starting to feel it. His house was five kilometres further. I passed the nursery on the corner of Gympie and Beams roads, and considered sleeping in their car park. The large displays of tiles were actually solar panels — that was how the area got its electricity. They were environmentalists here; Carseldine was a safe zone, a southern outpost deep in the north.

I turned up Beams Road. My legs were beginning to ache. My feet were going numb. Not far to go now. Thoughts of the region's politics, of spirits and vampires, werewolves, revolutions, all spun and whirled through my head violently, too fast to track. Politics was almost as tangible a force as wind gusting around me. My head spun, overburdened with these themes, these thoughts. I tried to shut it all out, but it was getting louder and incessant. I thought of my kung-fu instructor, an Asian man in his fifties, and of the vision of the giant panda in the trees at Paul's place — China. There had to be some wisdom I'd picked up that would suffice to clear my head of this noise.

I focused on one sentence as I walked. I repeated it with each step. I thought of nothing but the words, *I respect life*. It seemed the key lesson I hadn't yet learned, the reason for this punishment. I repeated the thought. *I respect life*, left, *I respect LIFE*, right, over and over. I clung to it, made it loud until it drowned out the other notions, the other ideas. *I respect life*. Left, right, left.

I paused at a roundabout, undecided. Paul's street was to the left, his home only a short walk away now. To the right was the Carseldine campus of the Queensland University of Technology, where I was still enrolled as a student. I could sleep at the campus, but the sinister forces following me should not be led there. It was sanctuary, but it was not impregnable. I headed there anyway, though mindful of the risk. A car passed — the secret police, looking for me. When it was out of sight I stepped into the university car park and sat cross-legged, waiting for something to happen.

The muscles in my legs were twitching from the walk and my feet throbbed. Intuition told me to leave this place; the tall brick houses opposite the campus looked menacing, little castles, well defended.

There was no choice: back up the road to Paul's. I passed a retirement home, where two young women sat talking in the car park beside their four-wheel drive. I sat across the road, watching them. They kept talking while they watched me back. I heard something along the lines of 'He broke the rules' and 'He's a bad dog'. Referring to my escape.

Paul's place was only a hundred metres away now. Bats flew from trees above me in a final warning sign that it wasn't safe there. I stepped through a spider web, which was a sign I had come to the right place after all; spiders, I'd heard, were the weavers of fate. I opened the side gate, stepped into the backyard, past the place where mosquitoes had swarmed over my legs the night before, and finally slumped down in a chair outside the back door to rest my sore feet. I'd made it. Paul's dog Tessa lay beside my chair. I'd spend the night here, guarding the house with her.

The hours passed. Some time between 4 and 5 am, Paul woke and came out the back door. He was surprised and relieved to see me. He said Mum had been phoning, she was worried sick. The hospital knew I was gone — they'd called around looking for me.

He told me to come inside, then folded out the sofa bed in the living room and got me a drink. I didn't know it at the time, but there was a sleeping pill crushed up in that drink. It took effect. I drifted away, despite the television. The escape was over.

In the morning my parents took me back. I slept most of the day, and when medication time came, I swallowed the pills. My feet and shins looked horrible, covered in mosquito bites and abrasions.

Already the hospital had ceased to seem like a Nazi death camp, didn't seem as menacing as it did when I was first brought in; still strange, still disorienting, but a place of rest, whatever else it was.

The other patients would sit in groups in the courtyard, talking in their strangely toneless voices. When I went out to smoke, it seemed from their conversations that they could see my thoughts, for they frequently commented on them. I tried to keep my mind as blank as I could. One of the guys kept saying loudly, 'The mind *will* wander.' He kept repeating it, as though to warn me about something.

We were allowed to walk around the hospital grounds during the day with far more freedom than the words 'mental hospital' perhaps suggests, although I was told there was a place where violent patients were taken, away from the rest of us. The hospital basically kept us busy and out of harm's way while the medication did its work. There was a recreation room that had arts and crafts activities, like a primary school classroom. Nurses oversaw this, suggesting projects if patients were around and in need of a way to kill time. There was a PlayStation in there too, also a room with a pool table, a gym and a cafeteria. I spent my time either smoking in the courtyard or sitting alone in my room, away from the other patients. Words did not make enough sense to spend the time reading, though I tried.

I kept to myself as much as possible, the plan being simply to ride it out until I could go home. A couple of the other patients approached me at times and tried to make conversation, but I was unresponsive. One of them warned me, 'We get all sorts in here. I mean, *all* sorts. Some guys who were in jail and said they were sick to get in here.'

The first few days I still felt like a frightened animal. The nurses would check up on me regularly, entering the room, making sure I was still alive. In response I armed myself with sharp pencils as I lay in bed. This feeling of threat quickly subsided when the nurses failed to attack.

Someone told me medication was pumped into the air conditioner's circulation. I think it was a method of discouraging patients from neglecting their oral medications — like saying you're getting the stuff through the air anyway, might as well take the pills. I was given physical check-ups, blood tests. These were terrifying; it's possible to conjure up many fanciful reasons for a doctor to pull out a syringe. After he tested me I felt angry and violated. I went into my room and threw some air swings at my reflection. The radio told me to settle down.

Cigarettes were the best way to pass time, which was how I got hooked again in earnest. Early in my stay I sat near a group of other patients in the courtyard, all smoking. I'd sat on the ground beyond the group, legs crossed, a gesture of humility, until they invited me to a chair, which they did almost immediately.

'What's your name?' they asked me.

'Will.'

One of them pointed at the septum ring I had in my nose and said, 'You ever get called a bull with a ring like that?'

I smiled. 'Not really.'

'Well, you're a big guy, you can take it.'

They introduced themselves. They seemed nice enough as I shook their hands. One called himself Ferret. He looked like a miniature biker, small, wiry, tattooed, with a mullet and goatee. He was crouched down on the floor on his haunches. When I shook his hand I looked him in the eye and sprang back, pulling my hand away, certain he was about to leap up and start clawing at my throat like an animal.

He had a friend, Greg, the one who'd kept repeating 'The mind will wander'. Greg was clean-shaven, taller than Ferret, thin and ragged-looking, with the face of a psycho: bony and wide-eyed. The earlier warning rang loud; I was sure these two were from jail. I made efforts to avoid them, but mealtimes were the complication. At mealtime everyone in our wing assembled in the dining room, a place of clanking, steaming metal carts, male nurses standing by, carefully watching the patients eat at long tables. Whenever Greg walked past I fully expected a knife in the back. I managed to psychically pre-empt his attacks; I'd lean forward at just the right moment, or hold up my cutlery in magical defence. The gestures were very subtle — the large male nurses would not have spotted anything amiss.

I was at the hospital for a week, but there was no real tracking of time there. All I wanted was to go home, and I realised I'd have to convince the doctors I was well enough for that to happen. So I followed the rules: got out of bed at the prescribed time, swallowed my pills, went to the dining room on time for meals (I'd have rather stayed in my room), went to bed at the prescribed time. When doctors interviewed me, I did my best to assure them I was miraculously cured.

Mum visited every day. She brought my CD player, my CDs and some books that I had asked for. From the CDs came a vast barrage of signals, mostly benign and encouraging; from the radio, when I dared listen to it, came commentary on my progress in a neutral, scientific tone. It seemed they were keeping track of me the way a documentary monitors the life and times of a wild animal.

STRANGE PLACES

I worried that the other patients would be jealous of my belongings, that I would have to fight someone. I did push-ups and practised martial arts moves in my room in preparation for such an event.

One of the days I was in hospital happened to be my twenty-second birthday. My parents, both my brothers and Paul's girlfriend came in that night to visit. They brought my guitar, as I had asked (I'd bought a cheap one after Dawn's visit, when rock-star fantasies had again loomed large), with a new set of strings. I still assumed I was to be some kind of musical prophet, so the spastic *plunk plink twang* of inept practice would become a constant soundtrack to those in rooms next to mine from then on. We sat in the dining hall, but the whole time I was conscious of the patients in the courtyard outside who could see in through the window. The sight of my guitar was, I was sure, going to provoke the attacks I'd been anticipating.

Another patient, a guy I'd spoken to on a couple of times, came in to say happy birthday. He was about my height, six foot five, with dark skin and a shaved head. I think his name was Jay. Rather than shake my hand, Jay grabbed me in a bear hug and leaned backwards, lifting me off the ground. This didn't seem like an assault to me, so I ran with it, and when he put me down everything was friendly. God knows what my family was thinking.

Paul, his girlfriend and I went to the courtyard to smoke. We sat on a bench in the eerie fluorescent-lit twilight. We were making small talk, puffing away, when Jay approached again and joined the conversation. He stood in front of Paul and said, 'I wanna show you something.' His words came out slurred and fast, always at the same low volume.

'All right,' Paul said.

Jay held up his first two fingers in a peace sign, with his thumb cocked to make an L. 'You know what that means?'

Paul didn't know.

'Means peace and love. You do it.' Paul held up his fingers in the same symbol. Jay then touched the tips of his fingers onto the tips of Paul's, and then began to push his hand forward towards Paul. 'Don't resist,' Jay said. He was speaking quietly. He continued to push his hand forward. 'Don't resist.'

Paul stepped back, not knowing how to respond. Jay was towering over him and, though generally harmless, was clearly not all there (nor did he precisely *look* harmless). Paul excused himself then walked back into the dining room. Can't say I blame him. Jay looked at me and said, 'I boomeranged it, didn't I?'

I knew what he meant.

Jay sat down next to Paul's girlfriend. He made small talk for a bit, then reached up and started stroking her hair, his face kind of slack — almost like a small child touching something because it's pretty. Paul's girlfriend fidgeted in her seat, clearly uncomfortable. 'Hey man,' I said, 'take it easy.'

Straight away Jay stopped, stood up, held up his *peace and love* sign, and walked away. He remained an enigma to me for the rest of my stay; a friend of sorts … but a friend to watch carefully. In a mental ward, I guess that's not uncommon.

Mum offered to take me shopping the next day to pick out a book and a CD or two for my birthday. The hospital said it was no problem, as long as she understood she would be legally responsible for me while we were gone. As we drove off, I hoped that maybe this was an escape. The floods were on their way again; perhaps we were going to get on board Uncle Richard's boat to avoid them.

We went to the huge mall in Chermside. Lesley met up with us for lunch. The mall's sights and sounds were very colourful and intense, almost too much to handle. The place was clearly a spaceship, taking the last of our species on a journey away from the doomed Earth. (The U2 song in heavy rotation then, 'Beautiful Day', had left me certain the world was doomed.) I stayed close to Mum and Lesley. The noise, the crowd — people all looking at me — it was massive. Sensory overload.

After we ate Mum took me to the bookshop and told me to pick something out. It was a long hard decision, rife with implications. Then Anthony Mundine's biography caught my eye. It had been dawning on me that I was Aboriginal, possibly from being housed with Jay and a couple of the other black guys in hospital. So I chose that book, and would spend a good part of the next week studying it, deciphering the codes, reading the signals. One signal vaguely, loosely hinted at writing. It was the first time in a very long while that the notion had sounded even briefly amid the other background noise in my head; since laying eyes on Dawn's bass guitar at the airport, I had believed my destiny lay with music.

To my disappointment Mum took me back to hospital, although it was a great relief to get away from the crowds of shoppers. I put my new possessions away and went out for a smoke, sitting at my usual spot just outside the door. Ferret, Greg and a few others were there. Ferret was staring at me for some reason. I looked down and saw that in his hand was a large bag of pot. He seemed to be showing it to me for some purpose I couldn't discern. I looked at the bag, then back up at him, not comprehending. He grinned at me in a way that may have been intended to say: 'Look what I got, brother — want some later?' At the time, I saw nothing but menace in his face.

Late that night a smoke alarm went off. This is a surreal event in a mental hospital. From my bed, I could hear patients in the other rooms panicking, with a wide variety of accompanying noises. The staff rushed around to reassure everyone that the sky wasn't falling while they investigated the alarm. I thought I knew what it was: Ferret's stash becoming smoke.

I opened my door and stood out in the hallway, and there he was, standing in the doorway of the room across from mine. We stared at each other for what seemed like a long time. Neither of us said anything. There was a threatening, ominous undertone there, tension promising to build to something. I turned away and went back to bed, but lay there uneasily. My door had no lock. I moved the wastepaper basket in front of the door so the noise of it falling over when the door opened would give me an extra couple of seconds to react and defend myself. I slept with pencils in my hands again for protection — they were sharp and could do real damage. But of course nothing happened.

* * *

The next day I was told that they were going to do some tests on me. I was taken to one of the large hospital buildings by the same bald nurse who I had fronted up to on my first day. He led me to a small room with what looked like a dentist's chair. The female nurse told me to sit down. I did, and the chair reclined.

Two models of human heads, made out of white foam, sat on the shelves on the wall opposite. One looked like a vampire; it had fangs drawn on it with black marker and yellow eyes coloured in. I stared at this, then looked up at my nurse and saw that she was a real, living vampire. She flashed me a smile, and two white needle-like fangs poked from her mouth, absolutely crystal clear, just for that one second. A blink later, she looked normal again. Somehow the fact didn't frighten me. If she was a vampire she would make me one as well. So be it — maybe there were worse things to be.

She made some markings on my scalp with a pencil, speaking reassuring words the whole while, apologising when I winced as the pencil tip dug in too hard. She attached electrodes to my head and flashed a light into my eyes. I think I slept during the remainder of the tests. When she was finished I asked her about the results. She smiled, and told me she thought it was 'a positive reading'. Had she fed on me? Was I now a vampire?

STRANGE PLACES

The tests had taken place during the lunch hour. The dining hall was empty when I got back, so for the first time I was able to eat on my own. At first I saw some significance in being alone in the dining room, something about the imminent launch of this alien spacecraft, masquerading as a hospital. I was enjoying the solitude when Jay walked in and sat opposite me. He asked for some of my lunch, so I let him pick out a couple of the cold ham slices from my plate. He said something curious: 'I had lunch already, I just never had a free one.' I nodded, understanding then, though I don't now. We shared the meal.

More time passed, more visits from my parents, my brothers, from Lesley. The whole experience of hospitalisation was so disorienting it meant a lot to have some sort of familiarity, even for a little while. Andrew showed up also — he graciously brought me in a supply of pornographic magazines. I remember asking him to bust me out of there, telling him I wanted nothing but freedom for my people. God knows what else I said.

He took it in his stride. All the while we were chatting, leaning against the wall of the main hospital building, I was certain that across the road the construction workers were all Chinese spies, that some had sniper rifles pointed right at us. I wasn't afraid, just tired of the whole thing.

All these notions and delusions now seemed fleeting, passing by like cars on the road, appearing then gone, maybe to return, maybe not. As the medication kicked in, they were broken into smaller pieces, gradually smashing that new jigsaw puzzle and revealing the true background behind.

After more interviews with doctors, I felt I had convinced them that I was well enough to return home. They spoke with my parents, and sure enough I only had a couple more days of hospital left. They said they could definitely use the spare bed. I spent the time reading Anthony Mundine's book, playing my guitar quietly, making some attempts to write poetry, though it made no sense at all. Meanwhile the medication was slowly but surely bringing me back to the real world, coaxing me step by step, like an infant learning to walk.

THIRTEEN

The day I was released from hospital, I sat out by the car park waiting for Mum to pick me up. I had my packed bag and my guitar beside me. While I waited, Ferret and another patient, a black man with tattoos on his arms down to the fingers, strolled past.

'You leaving, mate?' the black guy said.

I nodded. Then he said, 'I heard some guitar the other day. That was you?' I said yeah. 'You're pretty good,' he said (another little white lie). Ferret reached down and shook my hand. I gripped his hand without flinching — there seemed nothing threatening about him now; I supposed the black guy had some kind of magical power restraining him. They walked off. Soon my mother's car pulled up and it was time to go home.

We went to see a movie on the way back. My brother Justin was with us. Halfway through the film Justin and I agreed we just wanted to go home. I forget what the movie was called — the whole hour or so is a blur — but the huge screen was pouring out signals. I ended up riding home with Justin, who'd come in his own car, and singing along to the metal playing in his stereo. Screaming, in fact.

We stopped at the Foodstore I'd been busted stealing from, eight years before, so Justin could get some cigarettes. I saw a trucker walking from the store to his rig with a bottle of Coke. Again, that first signal echoed like fearful noise. He glanced over at me as I waited in the passenger seat. The euphoria of my freedom faded. That familiar old fear replaced it, just for a moment. Then it was gone.

My parents had paid my rent for the time I was in hospital, but I was in no state to function independently; I had to move out of that house and back home. The thought of being in the house with Robert (the cyborg!) was frightening, but I went back there with my folks to pack, and the aliens left us alone. We went home, and it was time again to start slowly piecing reality back together.

When I had my first episode, a case worker told me that if you had three episodes of psychosis you were technically schizophrenic. When a modicum of sanity returned this time, and the realisation that It Had

Happened Again, I didn't panic. It was just strike two. I wasn't schizophrenic. I'd just had two psychotic episodes, that was all. The condition wasn't necessarily permanent.

Over coffee and nicotine one morning, talking to Mum, I mentioned this — my relief that it could be worse. I remember the moment very clearly, sitting outside under the back patio, in the same spot Justin, Tony and I smoked all that pot, where I first thought there was a tap on the phone line.

'Second episode?' Mum responded bluntly. 'No, Will. You're schizophrenic.'

I said nothing for a second or two. Then I clenched my teeth and half yelled, half grunted, 'FUCK!'

Mum was apologetic. 'I'm sorry, I didn't mean to startle you with that.'

I was reeling. 'No, it's OK, but shit, I didn't think it was *that*, I thought it was just a second episode. Oh Christ. Are you sure? How do you know?' The doctors had told her, of course.

It was a horrible moment. Images of people going nuts, going on killing sprees came to me: all the stereotypical images that I felt I somehow — and this is the weird part — *ought* to live up to.

Schizophrenic … that word changed things. In my state of distress I called Warren and told him. I forget how the conversation went exactly, but as no stranger to bipolar himself, he was very reassuring. I remember one thing: 'There is no stigma attached anymore. You don't need to worry about that.' Boy did I need to hear that. They'd given me pills to take, I told him, which I suspected were placebos. 'Well, placebos always help,' he said. That, too.

What did that word mean, back then — schizophrenia? Absolute horror. Even the look and sound of the word made me wince (and still does, to an extent). It seems to suggest something foreign, a tentacled alien, an invading force, something inhuman. The kind of word spoken in lowered voices, whispered with faint awe. You can imagine people pointing to the lonely house at the end of the street, where the village hag lives, just a hunched silhouette by the window. 'Her? Don't go near that place. That's Mad Maud's house. They say she's got …'

Who would hire someone with that 'condition', as my mother always called it in gentle tones? What do you say on first dates? 'Oh, by the way …' How does one broach the subject when meeting the parents of one's new girlfriend (if one should be so lucky)? How does one fulfil one's potential and become, say, a lawyer, when one's doctor advises one to avoid 'stress', as 'stress' might send one careening over the edge again, just like a toke of a joint would (so you're told)? How does one get up early in the morning to study for one's law degree, when the pills make you sleep in so long? Can I not even have a fucking *beer* on New Year's now? Is that what it means? Am I always going to have these little signals? Even when ninety per cent of them stop, will that incessant, maddening ten per cent remain forever, a permanent fixture? What if — oh fuck! — what if I catch something *else*? What if I somehow 'contract' bipolar? Don't go telling me it's unlikely — I never thought I'd be *here*, either.

At first, there was fist-shaking at the heavens, there was petulance, there was anger without a real target to direct the anger at. Doctors and pills were the closest thing at hand. They seemed part of the problem. And sure, I was the one who sucked on that bong, but what the hell, how would you predict *this* outcome? Everyone else did it. And this is the kind of thing that only happens to other people. Isn't it?

First time around, it was a case of 'three years, then no more pills'. This time, the pills were here to stay, and there was no bullshitting about it. Life had changed — in fact, life seemed pretty much over. I made some attempt to write — to write this very account, in fact. I got some important details down, then quit in disgust. No more writing … with that nightly hammer-blow to the head and the hungover mornings, the results made it seem quite pointless (never mind that I'd written while medicated after Episode One). That particular dream had been pried away from me too, it seemed, and no, I was not cheerful about it.

I sat around the house doing nothing, just stewing about upcoming doctor's appointments and trying to kill time. I laughed bitterly to myself when the doctor tried to persuade me to do volunteer work to pass the time — no, thanks. My parents did not pressure me to find work; I was one of the lucky ones in that others were willing to support me. If not for them, I'd have lived on the streets, I'm sure, just like many others do. And on the streets there are drugs, and few reasons not to take them, and then you're on the merry-go-round, in and out of hospital for life.

I did not appreciate my relative good fortune — was wholly unaware of it, in fact, and perhaps not in the right frame to appreciate it. It would be a long time before I'd deal with the s-word in a mature way, or accept it as my cross to bear, or accept that there was no inherent reason why *I*, of all people, should be exempt from having a cross to bear. *If there's a way back to the real world, let it come to me. I've been through enough. I ain't moving.*

* * *

Recovery time. Rebuilding time. Slow, meandering time. Doctor once a week, case worker in between. Thumb-twiddling, doing nothing, oversleeping, overeating. Right now I was half stupid from the reintroduction to my old chum, the antipsychotic pill. Not Triazine this time, but something similar called Quezidone. Before long I was thirty-five kilos heavier.

Those were unhappy times. Depression set in kind of slowly, about the time I lost interest in writing stories and reading. I simply did nothing — at times I'd sit in my room, staring at the wall, and think: *Wow. I'm actually doing nothing. This is what it feels like to be doing absolutely nothing. How about that.*

I sold my guitar and a few other things and bought a computer, thinking that the online game I'd played when living with Robert, EverQuest, would be as good a way as any to kill the clock. Right I was, too — that game sucked away time like an obese vampire sucks blood. I got the internet connected and spent approximately an entire year of my life playing EQ, literally all day every day, often more than twenty-four hours in a stretch, entirely lost in the computerised fantasy world banally named 'Norrath'.

I made online friends from around the world: America, Sweden, Europe, even a fellow in Indonesia who ran a successful business, but told me he occasionally saw heads floating down the river when he crossed the bridge on his way to the office. With them I quested for loot, experience points, and glory. One day I bumped into Dawn, who still played the game, and who'd met a Canadian chap she was about to fly overseas to meet. I told her I'd been diagnosed schizophrenic. She said ouch, that sucked, but had news of her own: she'd been diagnosed bipolar when she got back to Melbourne.

Some people played EverQuest in healthy doses — a couple of hours after work, longer on weekends. But we were the hardcore addicts, people who sank serious time and emotion into their characters and conquests. And we left our real lives behind when we logged on. Many of us were unemployed, depressed people; others were students who were busily failing courses thanks to this game; others still were rich people who'd found the perfect alternative to work. Though many of us were unhappy people in reality, we were kings in Norrath, wealthy, powerful and admired. We killed dragons, battled through dungeons teeming with undead, had riches that made us the envy of other players.

But this required serious dedication. I stayed up all night in order to play in peak US time, and get my character to high levels in the fastest possible time. The radio, usually tuned to Triple J, was my companion — any songs I hear from that time take me right back to the cocoon, and sometimes I still miss its unhealthy comfort. I barely moved a muscle, except to go outside and smoke, or to replenish supplies of iced coffee and cigarettes at the service station. These were often midnight trips, leading the guy behind the counter to believe I was a shift worker, an illusion I gladly encouraged in order to gain his respect. I hardly saw sunlight beyond what crept through the blinds in the small spare room.

I didn't really shower much during this time, certainly not on a daily basis. My parents had to remind me most of the time, which I resented, and I didn't bother to hide my resentment. When reminded, I sometimes took a shower, sometimes didn't. Brushing teeth wasn't urgent either. It wasn't that I was trying to live dirty, it was just that the thought of taking a shower, changing my clothes, shaving, seldom occurred to me. As a heavy smoker, I didn't notice if I smelled. Not that it mattered anyway — Miss Right was hardly going to climb through the window at any moment, crying, 'Where is he? Where's that broke, mentally ill, overweight, uni dropout, computer game addict who lives with his parents I've been dreaming of?'

Andrew did his best to bring me out of this slump; he never stopped inviting me out to see a movie or play a social game of tennis or what have you. I usually refused. Too tired, I'd say. Doctor's appointment that day. Get off my back and stop trying to help me. I'm quite content to wallow.

The upshot was that the psychotic symptoms were dissipating. That happened relatively quickly. I avoided watching television, though, as I still got signals once in a while. When signals came from the radio — a sporadic occurrence — they were benign in nature. Like last time, the side effects of the antipsychotics seemed to be what was anchoring me here. At times it's hard to convince yourself that it's not better to be psychotic than overweight and mentally slow. Just once in a while, I'd tell my parents I'd taken my pills when in fact they were in the bin. This resistance was usually futile and didn't last long. If I heard a bump in the night, or a dog barking somewhere, and thought maybe I was about to start hearing voices, I would run straight for the meds.

The depression deepened. The long stretches of staying awake to play EverQuest didn't help; emotions and thoughts got a little skittled after a certain number of hours. I noticed that whenever I was feeling really down, an old habit would return from the days of battling psychosis without medication at the share-house. I'd shut my eyes and picture my wrist, gashed open and pouring blood, held up behind my closed eyes in defiance, like giving the surrounding world the finger. I knew all along how I would end it, if end it I must. I often found myself idly tracing a line down the veins on my wrist with my finger, sometimes before I even realised I was doing it.

I didn't succumb totally. Every now and then I'd devise exercise plans. I knew if I could get the weight off everything would change — I'd be able to go out and see friends, get laid once in a while. So I went for walks, I joined the gym and went swimming. It had worked the last time I'd tried it — but I'd also gone off the medication last time. Now, try as I might, the results just didn't come. I quit the exercise attempts quicker each time. All the while I told the doctors I was feeling fine, just to keep them off my back. I hated talking to them, loathed it.

My case worker at the time, David, tried in vain to give me advice on improving my situation. I had pretty much decided not to be receptive. I resented having to talk to him, and I got snappy and pissed off when my parents mentioned an upcoming meeting. Their patience throughout this time was commendable, but I still managed to push it to the limit. There's a reason my first novel is dedicated to them.

The worst of it soon came. After about a week of particularly deep depression, I decided to fuck the medication off altogether. I stayed awake for really long periods, drinking vast amounts of coffee. It felt like I was smarter, thinking clearer. I believed I was releasing my mind from the bonds of the pills. Of course, this ended in tears too.

FOURTEEN

I had a scare before the actual 'attempt'. The first time I really felt able and willing to kill myself came when my parents had gone out for the day. I worked myself up into a state of mania. Something triggered it — I went to the shop after days of not showering or changing my clothes and I think some young woman behind me in line at the service station made a comment about the smell, which, truth be told, must have been industrial strength. Or maybe I imagined it.

I got home, put my iced coffee in the fridge, and leaned on the counter. I'd been a *long* while without sleep by this stage. I replayed the incident, and started laughing.

I cackled with genuine glee at first. I laughed and I laughed and then, between heaves of laughter, I said aloud 'Hahaha, I couldn't give a fuck, couldn't give a fuck.' And then laughter became sobs. There was a touch of hysteria in those, too. I wandered around the house, wailing like a lost infant. I wasn't sure what to do. I went outside and sat at my smoke spot, crying real tears for the first time in quite a while. The image came right on cue, vivid: wrist held up, blood pouring.

I thought about the knife rack in the kitchen, big sharp knives. I toyed with the idea of going in right now, and slicing my wrists into shreds. I pictured myself walking in, grabbing the bread knife, and doing it, actually doing it. It would hurt but it would feel good. The dog came over and licked my foot to try and console me, then he wandered off, out of ideas. The world outside seemed suddenly colourless, like the life had drained out of everything. The wind blew strong and cold, but it, too, seemed lifeless.

And then very real fear hit me. They say that if you can still feel fear, you still want to live. But I knew that it was quite likely that soon I would lose control and I would actually do it. I'd never been there before; even in the shed at Paul's, after my knife-dance in the yard, I felt I had some control over my actions. Right then, at my smoke spot, it seemed I was about to lose my choice. I was about to actually run into the kitchen in a mania and butcher myself.

STRANGE PLACES

I stumbled inside and picked up the phone. I tried to call Andrew. His mother answered. I asked if he was there. She said no. She also asked if I was all right. I said yes. But if Andrew comes home please tell him to call me. It's important.

There was no one else to call. Paul. I dialled his number. It rang for a long time, but then he answered. 'Paul, it's me. I want to die.'

'Huh?'

'I want to kill myself. Can you come over?'

'What? Uh, shit. Um … shit. Yeah, I'm coming over. Wait there, OK?'

He came over. I told him what was wrong, which took some time. I said I was a fat blob, a waste of space. Look at me, for Christ's sake. Smell me. I told him I had no future, didn't want one — too much effort. I told him about the 'I gots no woman' blues, which problem wasn't likely to be fixed in the next decade at this rate. I told him about the side effects of the pills, the slowness, about things that had happened in the episodes which I hadn't told anyone else. He listened, tried to say the right things, but I was determined: my life was fucked.

Not wanting to leave me alone, he took me back to his place. On the way there he suggested I should write about all this crap. I told him I might, one day, and the idea resonated, but only for a while. I slept soundly that night. Things were better for a little while. The 'attempt', when it came, wasn't nearly so melodramatic.

I forget how much time elapsed between the scare and the attempt. Probably a couple of weeks. That whole period was a dull blur. For a little while I kept somewhat saner hours and took my pills. Then I stopped, for the same old reasons I'd stopped last time. When I had gone about four days without medication and about forty-eight hours without sleep I decided that today was the day. Time to die.

I wrote a suicide note. I've kept it, probably to keep me sober if for no other reason.

> I can't take this life. I can't take this world. I am sorry, so sorry it had to end like this. I never thought I would become the person that I am. I thought I would be something special. But I am an overweight schizophrenic with no prospects, and it goes downhill from here. I was going to write about my experience, as a last-resort attempt to deal with it. I couldn't even bring myself to do that much. I am a sack devoid of life.
>
> I think my time has come.

I could not have asked for better parents. Circumstance and unfortunate genes is what caused this.

I could not have asked for better brothers. You guys were there when I needed you, but I'm beyond reach now.

I could not have asked for better friends. Andrew, you tried and I thank you.

I can't make this note much longer. I am tired and want this over with. I am not in a state of psychosis or mania as I write this. I am calm and tired. I want it over with. I have hung on for Mum and Dad, can't do it anymore.

You all have a right to hate me for what I am doing. It is not your fault. It is partially mine, partially circumstance.

I love you all, please forgive me.

I will watch over you. BELIEVE THAT.

I WILL.

I was crying silently as I wrote that out on a page ripped from an exercise book. Then I went to take a shower. In the shower, I had an idea. I thought of a plan. My death wouldn't be meaningless after all. I had been telling the truth in the note, there was no mania as I wrote it. But a slight injection of mania came as I thought about things. I would get Them back, I decided. In that moment, They were there in the background, real, and every effort to paint some picture over the top of that psychotic reality was exposed as a sham: the picture behind was there all along, and by tearing away at the one on top — look! It was back. All else was willing self-deceit. So, I would make one last statement. One last act of revenge.

I dressed, then took my parents' car for a drive. I had a little cash on me. I went to the service station and looked for a glass Coke bottle. There were none; they'd been phased out. I cursed quietly, then drove to another service station. Same deal, no glass Coke bottles. I had planned to kill myself in a public place with a Coke bottle. Obviously that wasn't to be. I had to change tack. During the search I could feel the energy I needed to kill myself fading, and I worried that if I didn't do it soon I would back out.

Finally I found a glass Pepsi bottle, and grabbed a twelve-pack of Coke cans. The new plan was to slice my veins with a broken Pepsi bottle, then bleed all over the twelve-pack of Coke cans. Not perfect, but it would get the point across (whatever the, erm, 'point' would have been, exactly ...).

I bought the stuff, and winked up at the security camera as I left the shop. I drove, not really knowing where to go. Somewhere private, but where my death would get noticed. I ended up at my old high school, Dakabin. It was the mid-year school holidays and no one was there. I parked the car out front then hauled the drinks to the small area behind the tuckshop, smashing the Pepsi bottle on the way.

I sat and looked at the broken glass and my wrists. It wasn't like the last time I'd felt suicidal; I think a part of me knew it. I'd spent too much time that morning messing around, and now there was just a tiredness, no energy left to work myself into a suicidal state. I drew the glass across my wrist a few times, trying to talk myself into going through with it. I drew some blood, cutting both wrists, but not especially deeply. I poked the glass into the wounds, trying to go deeper. The blood came a bit stronger. Soon I had enough to add another touch to the scene. I wrote the word *Always* on the wall behind me in blood. The word had, since that 'first signal', given me a little jolt whenever I heard it. It was maddening, infuriating, that every time the word came out of someone's mouth I'd be reminded of the whole psychotic experience, condensed into that one little word. I tried to cut myself deeper.

It's ironic, how things panned out in the following minutes.

When I was three years old, younger perhaps, I was stung near the eye by a bee. It's my first memory. Ever since then I've had an intense phobia of wasps and bees. It's an irrational fear, of their colours, the buzzing sound they make when they get close to your ear. I especially hate and fear the huge orange hornets; when they come close to me, I run.

So I was sitting there in the spot I'd chosen to die, trying to convince myself to *actually* do it, when I looked up and saw big orange hornets, crawling over their nests made of hard mud. Oh, maybe six or seven of them. *Bzzzzz.*

I got the fuck out of there, pronto.

Home I went, not thinking much. When I got in, Mum and Dad were working in the yard. Mum saw me and came over, asking where I'd been — I'd taken the car without letting them know. I showed her my wrists, with the dried blood on them. The folks called the hospital, Caboolture this time, and off we went.

I arrived there feeling absolutely tired as hell and wanting nothing more than to get to bed. I spoke to a doctor, a risk assessor or something, and told her the moment had passed, my attempt wasn't much of an attempt, really. Scratches, that's all. It was agreed by one and all that hospital was the verdict. I didn't argue. They had beds.

I chatted to a couple more case workers — 'Please, for the love of God, let me sleep,' mostly — and finally had a room allocated. I wasn't delusional this time; I knew it was just a hospital, that the other patients were just patients.

I spent less than a week there. I wanted to get back home and get back to playing EverQuest — it occurred to me the next morning what a mistake I'd made, getting myself confined; I could have moved my dark elf warrior up another couple of levels during this time. My parents visited, of course, as did Andrew. I passed time reading fantasy novels and playing chess with another patient.

The Caboolture hospital was more laid back, less militaristic than Prince Charles. We weren't told specifically when to go to bed for one thing. The other patients seemed mostly to be depressed people who'd tried to hurt themselves. I saw one girl who'd tried my method, and she'd *meant* it. Huge deep scars covered both her wrists. She saw me looking at them and covered them up as though ashamed. My little cuts were nothing to those scars.

FIFTEEN

There seemed little way out of the rut: on that despicable medication, playing computer games, withdrawn from life. Medications are improving, however — mental patients of decades before would likely have done anything for a chance to take the medication I so detested. I was fortunate that a new one came out around then, and not a moment too soon.

My case worker David (to whom I will always be grateful) was well aware of my stagnancy from our sessions together, and he knew something had to change. He'd heard of the new medication, and maybe he'd seen others respond to it well. He suggested we try changing pills.

It was difficult to persuade my doctor of this course of action — to keep her off my back, I'd been telling her the whole while I was fine, when in fact I wasn't. David came with me to the doctor's appointment that day and watched nervously on as the doctor said, 'So, you have been responding well to this medicine. Why do you think you need to change?'

I grappled for a reason, without much luck, then inspiration struck: I muttered something about the current meds affecting my libido. The doctor's eyebrows raised, ever so slightly, then she shrugged and wrote me a new prescription.

I'm still not clear on what exactly snapped me out of things, apart from the change in medication. A few things stand out: Stephen King appeared in a dream and he shouted at me: 'Just fucking *write*! Just fucking *write*!' I'm of the belief there's more to dreams than little chemical plays of the mind, so it was one of the things that got me thinking about it again. Another thing was picking up the first of the Harry Potter books, not long after switching meds. It was a rare moment: I wanted a break from the game. I began reading, then ate up the first four books of the series over one weekend. That was a hint that there was life beyond the computer game.

On the new medication, side effects were dramatically fewer. I still kept bad hours and drank too much coffee, which didn't help things, but these pills somehow managed to combat what they call the 'negative symptoms' of the illness, the lethargy and depression. I moved out of home into a New Farm share-house with some friends I hadn't hung around with for years. This house would be physically identical to the house Jamie is living in when he's accosted by the clowns in my debut novel, *The Pilo Family Circus*.

There was suddenly a spring in my step, new energy, and writing again became the focus of all attention. I went back to uni, mainly to secure student payments from Centrelink, then spent most of my time either getting drunk in the city or writing.

Alcohol is not your friend, if you're not completely sane. Medication was a reasonably strong safety net, though it does not mix well with booze. I skirted close to outright alcoholism in this time, hampered only by a lack of money; had I adequate funds, I may never have left the nightclubs. Sometimes I'd hit the town with only ten bucks in my wallet, then strike up a conversation with someone in the hope they'd buy me a beer. It often worked. Then there were people who couldn't quite finish their beers — 'You going to drink that?'

Still keeping weird hours, I'd drink after a long period of sleep deprivation, then stagger home from the pubs and clubs just before dawn, certain people were following with bad intentions. I had a Maglite torch in my bag, a heavy metal torch cum club favoured by security guards, which I'd hold out in the open and rattle against wire fences as I passed to scare these invisible pursuers away. Then, swallow the pills, lights out, trying to believe that the streetlight visible through the bedroom window was just a streetlight and not some alien spy device.

Throughout this time, though, I wrote. That is the great secret trick beginning writers sometimes struggle with: actually sitting your backside there at the keyboard or notebook and doing your daily shift. I did short stories at first to limber up the muscles, then before long out came a novel-length manuscript. It was done in four fevered weeks, a somewhat originally constructed fantasy which, if read by anyone, would at best 'show promise' (though my proofreaders were full of praise). At seventy-thousand words, the first manuscript was a major psychological breakthrough.

Even though it will never be published, that effort got some key things right, things I was hardly conscious of during the act of writing it. The main breakthrough for me was learning to manage multiple characters — all the other elements of a good novel (pacing, plot and so on), were handled well, but by instinct, not conscious design. The plot fitted neatly, action and revelation were correctly paced to build suspense, and characters were developed — not in the way a pro would do it, but in a less amateurish fashion than you'd get from most first-timers. I did not realise that I was doing these things; I was just writing a long story, and doing it in the fashion of stories I liked reading.

This is not to say the writing itself was anywhere near publishable yet. The formula I hit on breaks novel-writing down into two basic tasks: draft one establishes *content* (what happens, who does what, so on) and subsequent drafts establish *delivery* of the content (that is, polishing the writing.)

I had only mastered the content part at this stage of the apprenticeship; that I had done so intuitively was a good sign, but the technicalities of the writing were far short of the standard needed. It takes multiple subsequent drafts to get the writing where you want it; back then, my second draft consisted of a skim-edit over the course of a week — and running the spell-checker, of course.

However, at the time I thought my manuscript was a masterpiece. I got drunk in celebration, staggering home in the morning, proudly telling strangers on their way to work that I'd just finished my first novel. I assume they realised I meant writing one, not reading one — from my drunken, bleary, red-eyed stagger, it could have gone either way.

STRANGE PLACES

Since I didn't have a printer, I took a disk to a copy centre up the road and paid twenty dollars to get it printed. Twenty dollars was a fair slice of my beer money — this was serious sacrifice and dedication. At home I noticed the small army of typos and mistakes, fixed them, paid another twenty dollars, then noticed yet more mistakes ...

I'd assumed that all you really had to do was write a story of sufficient word-length, and then hey presto, the rest would fall into place; after all, making the word-length was the hard part. Then you'd be an author, paid squillions, admired by all. Submitting this thing, this dog's breakfast of a manuscript, wasn't likely to get more than a wry smile from any agent or publisher. Nonetheless, I posted it off to a handful of publishers, certain the offers would be rolling in soon. The cover letter that went with it was long-winded and informed the recipient I'd written that first book in just five weeks, so I'd be able to churn out probably six, seven per year.

I immediately began work on the next one, a comic fantasy set partly in life as we know it, partly inside the mind of a character who joins a religious cult. I'd made a landscape of the fellow's brain, and characters out of various parts of his mind: each emotion, his logical faculties, his libido, the one in charge of his dreams, and so on. When the protagonist joins the cult, a slimy con man takes the Department of Logic by force. The internal characters band together to try and pull their dense host out of trouble.

The result was a little tame and cutesy for my tastes, but still a step closer to publishability. The main thing was reaffirming the formula I'd hit on with the previous manuscript. It began with deciding on a setting: this world, or a fantasy world, completely cut off from ours? Or a hidden other world which met or collided with ours? Then came sketches of characters, brainstorming of plot possibilities, but not too much outlining at the outset — characters were to lead the story around. Plot possibilities were to be chosen from if things stalled.

The feeling of finishing a novel-length story is one of inertia; so much willpower, energy and thought, both conscious and subconscious, have been directed to the task, it's like the car you've been driving has pulled to a sudden halt, and you're still lurching forward, seatbelt across your guts.

We had an interesting collection of people in that house. Quite often we were all boozed up, but life was vibrant. One of my roomies sold a little hooter, so customers were frequently visiting and hanging around in the living room

STRANGE PLACES

as their goods were chopped up and bagged. They weren't seedy types at all, they were always friendly and well dressed.

Still, too much time in my cocoon away from people meant I had a few things to rediscover about socialising and co-habiting. I was not an ideal roommate — I used other people's towels, occasionally flipped my lid, didn't pick up on basic etiquette points. I was still in a strange head space then, ping-ponging between sleep deprivation, drunkenness and the lethargy of hangovers made worse by medication that should not have been mixed with alcohol. I almost got in a punch-up with my good friend Dan over a stupid misunderstanding during a drinking session. If I had something to say to my roommates, I'd write some awful abstract poem, then Blu-Tack it to the dining room wall upstairs. After a few months they asked me to move out.

I moved into a little apartment in Strathpine, on my own. That was a good way for me to live, just then — no one to bother me, no one to bother. My own hours, my own mess, and no longer just a short walk from the pubs and nightclubs of the city. Mum dropped by now and then to help clean the place up and make sure I had some semblance of vegetable matter in the fridge. I hit second-hand book shops, stocking up on paperbacks. I bought a copy of *The Australian Writer's Marketplace*. All was in readiness: I had my little nest, cut off from the world. Welfare paid the rent, with a little help from my parents, who could not easily afford it. Money was too tight for any fun, but no matter, for it was time to cut the shit and get busy.

SIXTEEN

This was the period in which I'd write my breakthrough novel. It was a productive little apartment, one of four old brick units on a block not quite built for units, with two bedrooms, a weak shower and an oven whose door didn't shut properly. Due to the block's irregular shape, the neighbours were very close. Standing on the front balcony, and looking left to right, they were: a pool store, an Indian goods store, a paint shop, a bald old man missing several fingers named Frank. To Frank's immediate left was a Cash Converters. This meant all the local burglars and drug fiends were tiptoeing past my place to sell their stolen bounty, a fact you couldn't help but be acutely conscious of. One of the other three units invariably housed a young couple with a penchant for domestic violence (at least three such couples lived in that flat while I was there).

Throughout these years I seldom left the house, especially early on — only to play indoor cricket or to go to uni (one subject per week, enough to keep student welfare payments), and, later, to work at a casual job Paul scored me at a law firm in the city.

Those few years were a continuous and exhausting burst of writing. Again, the lengthy edit/rewrite process was neglected; instead, I just mined novels and stories raw, to be refined later (though they seemed refined already to my untrained eye). Short stories were plentiful; my strategy for publication was to score wins in a whole bunch of short-story competitions. That way, I'd have an impressive cover-letter to send with the novels. (Since the form rejection letters had rolled in for my first couple of manuscripts, it began to dawn on me that being published wasn't going to take just reaching the word-length; submitting well, it seemed, was as important as writing well.)

From *The Writer's Marketplace*, I typed out a list of competitions and stuck it to the wall. I needed to send a story away every couple of weeks, though the entry fees and postage pressured my tight budget. In addition, I had to do several thousand words per day of whichever novel was currently in progress, and keep up a heavy reading regimen. There weren't enough hours in the day to do all this, so I simply extended the day, keeping the kind of hours I'd kept when playing EverQuest.

My third novel, called *Oddity*, was another affirmation of the multi-character formula. It was a strange mix of horror and comedy, this time set in a world totally cut off from ours. I thought I was making some kind of political point, too, but as my views were informed more by the psychotic period than by reality, as an allegory it failed resoundingly. Some of the characters, however, were really memorable, and it pains me that they'll never see the light of day. At just over eighty thousand it was also a new record word-length.

After this, I tried something different, a smaller novel of straight horror called *Rehab*. In it, a junkie overdoses on heroin and winds up comatose. I thought that comatose people could on some level still be aware, though what they perceived may not be pleasant. For instance, my unconscious protagonist smells pine disinfectant in a hospital, which translates in his comatose world to an artificial-looking pine forest, through which he travels, encountering all kinds of horrors. Nurses tending to his comatose body are likewise presented as distortions in his secret nightmarish life. The things they do to his body — inserting a catheter tube, for instance — become disproportionately horrible events in his private little hell. He meets up with other comatose people in this false universe. The plot was a noir parody of *The Wizard of Oz*, though absolutely straight-faced.

The tone of this one was very different to the others, much darker, and I was turned off by the lack of humour — there was zero comic relief. I sent it to a couple of publishers, but never really got behind it (not that it was sufficiently redrafted to be publishable anyway). Meanwhile, the clock was ticking, years were passing, and I began to wonder just how long it was going to take to break through. Could I keep it up till age thirty? That had been the plan. Surely that would be long enough, if I kept producing five thousand words per day. But it was just starting to dawn on me that being broke and living this insulated life wasn't in any way romantic, that this was time I wouldn't get back, time in which others were getting degrees or jobs or savings. What if I hadn't made it by thirty? Then what? Go back to law school? And was I supposed to be alone this whole time? Could that be done, or would bitterness consume me? Those questions began to gnaw at me in a most unpleasant way.

For the next project, I wanted to return to a third-person multi-character fantasy/comedic novel, more like *Oddity* had been, though perhaps somewhat darker than that tale, though not quite as dark as *Rehab*. I began scouting for ideas in a brainstorming session that would prove somewhat fateful. I'd decided on a mixed-world setting: beginning in our world, then entering another. That kind of fantasy was what I was most into reading at the time — Neil Gaiman did it beautifully in *Neverwhere*, and Jasper Fforde, though he's more a satirist than a fantasy writer, did a nice world-blending trick in his Thursday Next books. And of course there are the Harry Potter books, which bullseyed the mixing of worlds with a cheeky audacity like not much else has before or since.

A circus seemed like the kind of setting I was after; it made characterisation easier to start with, knowing there were certain roles to fill. You needed clowns, of course, and acrobats, and you needed a proprietor or two. You needed a freak show, a fortune teller, a magician, then a large pool of miscellaneous characters, from which other significant players could be drawn if needed, like dwarfs and gypsies.

All this was like filling in blanks. I drew the clowns first up and thought the results could be fun to play around with. The drawings told me a little about each character. For example, they told me Gonko wore magic pants, and that from his pockets he could pluck whatever he needed in an emergency. (Gonko, the clown boss, is the character people tell me is their favourite, along with Kurt Pilo, the ghoulish circus proprietor.) I was especially fond of Goshy the clown — for some reason his drawing really creeped me out. I liked the idea of a major character not speaking a single word of intelligible dialogue, too, despite being quite vocal.

With some more drawings and conceptualisation, including the traditional fantasy-world map, I had my setting. I Blu-Tacked it all to the walls above the computer, a practice I'd discovered made it easier to keep track of multiple characters for plotting purposes. It made it feel like I was working with tools, combining things already there, rather than plucking things from the ether.

Now I needed a protagonist from the real world, and a way to connect our world to the circus. Basing characters on real people was not something I'd done before, nor something I'll do again. But my best friend Andrew, who maybe didn't think this thing would ever actually end up published and purchasable by his friends and acquaintances, said no problemo when I asked if I could cast him in the story. So in he went: share-house, job, character traits, flaws and all. Three months later, my rough draft was finished, the final ten thousand words done in one long caffeinated sitting.

Because of the book's plot, interviewers have asked if *Circus* is autobiographical. In it, Jamie is hassled by some unusual clowns — they appear out of nowhere at his workplace, at his home, in his dreams. They tell him he's auditioning for the circus, and it's obvious a messy end awaits if he fails. He passes his audition. He's kidnapped, taken to a little netherworld just next door to hell, where there exists a secret circus filled with monstrous, ghoulish characters. People from our world are lured there and their souls are taken. Meanwhile, the bickering and infighting between circus personnel is like a churning sea of nastiness, and Jamie drops right in, headfirst.

To bring out the clown personality within him, the clowns give him some magic white face paint. When he wears it, there's a Jekyll-and-Hyde effect, and out comes JJ the clown, a most unpleasant chap who ever so slightly resembles Andrew when he's had one too many brews. The two personalities end up at war — JJ's enraged that Jamie won't surrender complete control of the body they share, and Jamie, of course, wants to get the hell out of the circus, maybe even shut the evil enterprise down, if possible.

This split personality may be why some people ask if the face paint is meant to represent schizophrenia. That wasn't the intention. I was worried at the time of writing that my friend Andrew was getting a bit too boozy for his own good — at that New Farm house, which he'd moved into, alcohol was the staple diet.

Of course, it's not hard to spot some emerging themes in the description of these stories: a character transported to another reality, often far less pleasant, by forces beyond his control, then the ensuing battle to get back to the reality he'd known before. I could tell you this has nothing to do with mental illness; it's never a conscious choice when writing these stories, they just work out that way. But it's like they say: believe the story, not the storyteller.

When I finished *The Pilo Family Circus* I had no sense that I'd done something significant. To me, it was just manuscript number five, a natural progression from the others, and a new word-count record at one hundred and twenty thousand. I was pleased with the results, but not over the moon by any stretch. The characterisations seemed OK, though often less memorable than in *Oddity*. There seemed fewer real belly laughs, though maybe as a dark fantasy it was a stronger, more rounded effort. The writing was rough, still, and a long way from being the relatively polished draft I'd submit. Some part of me recognised this — I kept it away from the postbox, for now. I began rewriting one of the earlier works, while still churning out short stories, and thinking about the next novel.

It would be a couple of years before *Circus* would become a book — the first draft was written in 2004, the book was published in 2006 — and it's hard to find entertaining ways to describe how that couple of years were spent. During that period, I came close to throwing in the towel and doing other things with my life. Strathpine, on the north side of Brisbane, does not seem like a launching pad from which big things are possible, and that relentless normality kind of rubs off on you and is hard to deny. Had I been saner — keeping regular hours and forgoing those feverish writing sessions — I may have listened to the sensible voice inside which told me to stop all this foolishness and try a normal career.

Picture someone up very late in a lonely little brick apartment, sitting at a computer, iced coffee open beside him, tapping away below sketches Blu-Tacked to nicotine-stained walls. Or he's reading — maybe Tristan Egolf's *Lord of the Barnyard* for the fifth or sixth time, or a Stephen King paperback, or John Kennedy Toole's *Confederacy of Dunces* — in a worn recliner whose seat has sunk in, making it comfy but hard to stand up again. There's an ashtray balanced on one arm of it, packed to the brim with grey ash, spilling over the side. There are empty plastic iced coffee bottles and dirty coffee cups piled up everywhere. Ash is spilled in the cracks between letters on the keyboard. There are books and sheets of paper scattered all over the place. It's a mess.

He has been awake a long time, most likely. He thinks he's escaping the effects of the medication by doing this — yes, even the improved medication has some unpleasant side effects — but in reality, the hangover feeling every morning has more to do with the hours he keeps than medication. He's been up for maybe forty hours this time — a long day even by these odd standards, but not uncommon. He's feverish, not thinking right, closer to psychotic than a doctor would like, but in a controlled way; sleep and pills will bring things back to normal. He tries to use the unusual thoughts as a source of ideas.

Sleep time, at last, sleep. But that will be a problem. He's got a lot of caffeine in his system, many toxins from cigarettes. Chances are it's broad daylight, too, and that there's plenty of noise; cars starting in the garage directly below the flat, crows bawling, garbage trucks emptying industrial bins in the paint shop car park just next door.

When he takes his medication and tries to drift off, it won't be easy. Every time, it happens: he will lie there and his mind will go to strange, unpleasant places. There will be an irresistible urge to get up and eat something, the appetite insatiable (scooping leftovers with bare hands from bowl to mouth, crouched before the fridge, swaying on haunches, barely conscious). Lying in bed, he will become certain spiders are crawling all over him, and he will sometimes feel pain in his feet, certain they are biting. There will be a feeling like electric sparks being pressed into his lower back; his legs will twitch and stiffen, kicking out on their own. When he gets up to piss or eat, his heart will palpitate, and he will feel certain at times he's about to die, *this very second*. Sometimes at night he will see what looks like electricity pulsing through the room, and this eerie light will wake him up.

Turning on the hall light and leaving the door open is a little help at first, but not for long. This old apartment may be haunted. One evening, after a rare lapse into alcohol, combined with lack of sleep, he sees the silhouette of a woman standing in his bedroom doorway, looking in. He blinks and she's gone as his heart beats very fast indeed.

Sleep is an epic, hellish struggle, every time, but for two years I don't cotton on that caffeine is the problem. Strangest of all, sleep is so deep when it comes, and so long — fourteen, eighteen, twenty hours, depending on how long I'd been awake — that I practically forget the nightly hell when I wake, forget it completely until it's bedtime again, many, many hours later. This unpleasantness I blame on the medication, and I consider reducing the dosage; but I consider a relapse, consider being put on the old meds again as a consequence, recall life on Triazine, and

Quezidone, and vow not to go back there no matter what. Psychosis would be preferable. Suicide would be preferable.

Worried about cancer from my cigarette habit I down vitamin pills and fish oil tablets with each meal. In the kitchen, bills are piled up, ignored until the last possible second. It's not real poverty when there are parents willing to spot you fifty dollars now and then, but the rent's gone up again, and it's not exactly luxury either.

The neighbours in unit two are loud and violent. Glass breaks at night, there are shouted obscenities to the backdrop of rap music, Eminem and 50 Cent. Her screams, his shouts, sometimes she the apparent aggressor until he can take no more and slaps her one. The clink of bottles being unpacked from their car in the afternoon is a sure precursor to a fight that night.

When my welfare payment goes into the bank, it is a day of celebration. I go across the road to the supermarket, stocking up on iced coffee and buying a carton of smokes. With these two things I can function; without them, no writing gets done. Fortnights of poor management sometimes leave me short of cigarette money; my watch has been pawned to Cash Converters for twenty dollars many times, likewise my little stereo, then bought back on pay day. Other times, I'll endure the wait, and hang around the ATM at five in the morning, or earlier, waiting for the payment to clear. If the payment's late, I'm in for a rough morning of withdrawal and cravings.

Meanwhile, also up on the wall, there are dates of upcoming short-story competitions. Sometimes postage costs and entry fees mean being short of addiction money, but that's just too bad. I go through the short stories, dozens of them, mostly no good, and try to work out which ones I'll send where, which ones deserve more attention, which ones are just wing-and-a-prayer entries. I've usually been up a while when I head across the road to the post office with a bunch of envelopes to get money orders for entry fees. The sunlight seems far too bright. My footsteps feel unsteady, I speak too quickly, have had too much coffee again, scare people by accident — head shaved, face not, eyes red, I look like a crim. Old people try not to make eye contact, people walk fast to get out of the way. It's kind of depressing.

I feel some strange satisfaction as the envelopes drop into the postbox, like a fisherman casting lines in water.

Then, of course, I check the mail religiously. I've sent off manuscripts too, here and there, in bursts. It takes weeks or months or most of a year to hear back. I've sent them to agents, to publishers, but the works are not ready, not close to being ready; the writing's too sloppy, not carefully enough edited. Manuscript number two, *Inside Out*, will eventually see both an agent and a publisher get back in touch, but, agonisingly, lead to nothing.

I'm thinking of life post-publication, imagining, wrongly, that it will be like getting the key to some utopian life where all problems — money, loneliness, addictions, being trapped in this fucking godawful little apartment whose oven door won't shut — will be magically solved. I'm envisioning it: one more year, then I'm there. One more manuscript, then I'm there. Learning more about writing with each manuscript; hang in there. Getting better each time; hang in there. By Christ, if it takes me fifteen, I'll write fifteen. I'm telling myself, *My advantage is* time. *My competition, the other writers on the slush pile, have jobs; I don't. I'm therefore broke and trapped here, but I'm tough enough to cop that, complaints notwithstanding. I'll beat them to it because I'll work harder. I'll work longer. Just keep it up till I'm thirty.*

It's sprinting a marathon, but really, where else am I headed? I've put myself in a position of do or die, knowingly cornered myself. Five thousand words in a day — in a stretch of wakefulness, more accurately — is pleasing. Three thousand words is acceptable, but not great. Two thousand is not good enough. Words of new content are considered — mistakenly — to be of greater value than rewritten content; I'm yet to learn the crucial importance of editing and revising. I'm yet to read John Gardner's *The Art of Fiction*, which will eventually correct so many errors and set me straight on so many points. For now, working methods are scattergun: do so many stories and there will be some good ones hitting their target, rather than carefully aiming, crafting one at a time and getting it right. Hence, there are half a dozen good stories and many, many sub-par. It's the same with the novels.

In between drafts of manuscripts I'll anxiously try to work out what the next project should be. Rewrite the *Circus*? Nah ... *Inside Out*'s due for reworking, I've got a feeling about that one. Or maybe short stories for a couple of weeks. Begin a new novel maybe? It's a two- or three-month commitment; I stew and sweat on it.

The greatest days are when there's mail, and in the mail are notifications from competitions, saying I've made a shortlist. It's not a win, but it's something. The first time this happens, it is affirmation of the whole ambition, wind in my sails. It staves off ideas of giving up; it's another promise of that utopian key. It's coming, that key, keep going. Run. The less-than-great days are when results come of a competition without my name on the shortlist or among the commendable mentions.

For the five or six certificates of congratulations for making shortlists, I buy cheap frames from Crazy Clarks, Blu-Tacking them to the wall, where they often fall down with a crash in the middle of the night.

Most days there's no mail but bills.

A crazy old woman has moved into unit four. Strange sounds come through the walls. She has a small child and often screams at him; I wonder if I should call the cops. When the screaming happens at midnight, and I hear the words 'I'll kill you' growled through clenched teeth, followed by the *thump-thump-thump* of someone sprinting madly through the apartment, I do call the cops.

From my bedroom, I hear them kick down the door and overhear: 'Yeah she's in here. Something's wrong. There's no furniture, no food or anything. Get the kid out, get the kid out.' A week later the crazy old woman is lurking around the letterbox, and she gives me a furtive, almost apologetic look, then she's never seen again.

The people in unit two are fighting, as they often do. Glass breaks. Screams. Next day the male comes over and asks if he can run a power cord through my laundry power point. 'The bastards've cut off my power,' he explains. He's standing in the doorway, wiry, no shirt, tattooed, shaved head, squaring his shoulders, trying to intimidate. One of his front teeth is chipped so it's triangular — my eyes can't leave this nicotine-stained triangular tooth. I do not like the way I stand out so visibly in a room of people on most days, but at times like this I'm glad to be six foot five. I'm also glad my cricket bat is beside the door, and I'm willing to use it ... by Christ, I'm willing to use it. I tell him politely that power costs money and I don't have much of that — nothing personal. He offers to pay, but doesn't have the money on him right now, of course ...

Without television to distract them there's more fighting that night as they bash and thump in headlocks against the aluminium fence by the block's driveway, the guy and a male friend of his who has come over for cones. The new neighbour from unit four comes out to break it up, screaming at them that he has 'a baby daughter up there, and she's scared,' then he keeps on screaming, threatening, himself eventually making more noise, and for longer, than the fighting people were.

The time lurches by, sometimes crawling, sometimes sprinting when I'm not watching. The hours I keep make it very hard to keep track of time; sometimes a week seems to pass in a day, sometimes memories of last month seem years old. Some days — the day before the welfare hits the bank — seem never to end. I'm working on *The Pilo Family Circus* again, the manuscript I haven't submitted yet, wanting to get this one right this time. It's rewrite number three or four. I'm reading *The Art of Fiction*, and it's a revelation; I've not been going about this job in the best way. I'm making common mistakes, there's not enough intense scrutiny of each sentence — not just its meaning, but its structure, the sound, rhythm and melody of words.

Rent's going up. One hundred and seventy dollars a week. When I first moved in, it was one hundred and ten. Ah, the 'property boom' … let the good times roll.

The crows parked on the roof next door are driving me up the fucking walls. They go non-stop, all day, *caw, caw, caw*, so loud, so very loud. There's a family of geese in the yard next door too, and one particular goose is giving me an ulcer; *rark, rark, rark*, as loud as a car horn through the bedroom window. I have never hated an animal until this moment. I want to kill it, I really do. Some days it makes that noise every five minutes.

Then there's the paint shop just over the side fence — every morning, nice and early, CLANG BOOM CLANG as they unchain the tin ladders and pack them onto utes. I get pleasure occasionally from staring out through the blinds as these tradesmen make this racket; then they sense themselves being *watched*, and look about nervously. Plans for vengeance are made but never acted on. I'm tempted to charge out there one morning with the cricket bat, screaming threats. I believe it would get results. These noises, more than anything, are making me feel trapped in this hot little brick box, wearing me down and making me want out of here, out of this situation, to find life's Plan B. This is jail.

Things are seeming bleak now. I've heard back from an agent about *Inside Out*; they've requested the full manuscript to read. From a major publisher, I get an email, the email's title, *Publishing Proposal*. In these moments, I think I've made it, think I'm *there*, and drop to my knees to say prayers of thanks — but I'm not there. I've heard about how manuscripts have to go through many, many hurdles from the initial contact, but I assumed, of course, I'd be an exception to the rule. I'm therefore shocked and saddened when I find I'm not.

There was a time when this would spur me on. Not anymore. I don't think: *I got close! How encouraging.* I think: *I am fucking sick of this. How long can I keep this up?*

There are other low moments. Once, I send *Oddity* to a British publisher, whose details a well-meaning relative passed on to me. In the mail I get a fancy-looking letter, which tells me the company would be 'delighted to offer a publishing contract for *Oddity*, followed by much praise of the manuscript. I lap it up. My heart races. I whoop and make a fist and punch the air. I'm already on the phone, calling my family to break the news.

On the phone, I read the letter out loud, right up to the part where it says all they need is two thousand pounds … Oh.

When the agent gets back in touch about *Inside Out*, she says it reminds her of Terry Pratchett, but that it may need some work. She mentions a manuscript assessment service, run by a published author, who reads a manuscript in full and offers detailed advice on its publishability, or otherwise. They send a report, and a positive report can be a great way to get people in the biz to look at your stuff more closely. There are dodgy ones out there, who will happily write a five-hundred-dollar fan letter, but this service has a good rep.

I send *Inside Out*. Finding the money for it — several hundred dollars — is not easy. An overdraft account helps.

Many weeks pass before I get the report back, saying *Inside Out* has potential but is not up to scratch yet, and listing the reasons why. I'm gutted, and debate with the report, argue against it, conceding some points but not others, only later to look at it clear-headed and realise the report is pretty much on the money. I add another rewrite to the to-do list, right after I've completed the current task, which is rewriting *Circus*.

When I'm done, I dip into the overdraft for another five-hundred bucks to send *Circus* to the same assessor. When I do, it occurs to me I'm burned out and in sore need of a vacation, or at the very least A change of scenery. I can't afford either. I finish the *Inside Out* rewrite in a few weeks, doing a frantic but not especially thorough job. I dip into the overdraft for yet another five hundred or so, and send it to the same assessor, still waiting to get the *Circus* report back.

What does a fellow do if a holiday isn't possible? Online video games, of course. When times are tough, that comfortable time spent cocooned playing EverQuest seems to me to be a fond, dear memory, with none of the underlying unhappiness of that time; it's the easiness I remember, the lack of effort required. These days, my friends are all into World of Warcraft. I buy a copy and some computer upgrades with what's left of the overdraft money. My character, an undead warlock, is at level 60 within a month, because I do nothing else with my time … nothing at all.

I have a feeling of dread when the *Circus* report arrives in the mail. Due to large volumes of submissions, it's taken them longer to get it back to me than the usual five weeks. Taking the thick yellow envelope from the letterbox, I immediately recall all the story's flaws and shortcomings, and for a day or two I don't even open it. Too much is riding on this. I don't have it in me to go back to the drawing board right now; I'm spent. I play World of Warcraft and try to forget about the thick yellow envelope.

When I open it, I read it and literally cannot believe my eyes. Is this a joke? I am numb. I shake my head. My hands may even be shaking a little as I place the report carefully in a drawer and don't touch it again for two weeks or more. I don't dare. What if it has somehow changed?

SEVENTEEN

Towards the end of 2005, Mum mentioned a new ABC competition, an award for 'an original unpublished fiction manuscript by an Australian resident aged 18 years or over'. She'd heard about it on the radio.

I'd begun rewriting *Circus* with the changes suggested by the assessor; while the report was very favourable, and seemed to indicate publication was likely, there were still a few things to finetune. The pessimist within took over the reins again, too, and whispered in my ear that this changed nothing; I was still in this goddamned apartment, after all.

But I put World of Warcraft aside and gave *Circus* the finetune it needed. I was busy enough not to worry too much when the second report for *Inside Out* came back, saying that despite the work done, it was still a case of 'close but no cigar'. At that point I'd had enough of working on it and decided it was time to bury the sucker for good; enough time had been wasted on it, and it had contributed enough to my current feeling of burnout. I haven't touched it since and don't intend to.

The manuscript of *Circus* I sent to the competition hadn't yet incorporated the changes suggested by the report, so it was not with a great deal of confidence that I took it to the post office on the day before the deadline, slid it into a large express envelope (with a twenty-dollar money order for the entry fee), and dropped it into the postbox about fifteen minutes before the day's mail pickup. I didn't think much about the competition after that, having already entered dozens of competitions for no result. *Hell, it'd be nice to make the shortlist*, I figured.

I also posted a sample of the manuscript to some literary agents, with a much more polished cover letter, following the formula outlined in Bob Mayer's *The Novel Writer's Toolkit* (which I also recommend). A sample is all agents usually ask for at first. If they want the rest after reading it, they'll let you know. An agent can tell, often after a page, whether or not a manuscript will be of interest. (Some writers have therefore mastered the art of a good first three pages with nothing of interest to follow.)

The odds are always, always slim. The competition is fierce, more so since the rise of creative writing courses, and a pitifully small number of books per year are published by new authors. In my favour, this time, I had a positive assessment report from a reputable assessment service to send with my work. But that was all. Everyone else — my brother Paul for one — was more confident about my chances this time than I was. The only clue I had that things might change was a dream in which someone told me in a dead-serious voice: 'They're considering you for an award.' As in, get ready.

Don't taunt me. It was back to World of Warcraft and nothing else. I was burned out, sick of it all. The conditions at the flat had worn me down. If *Circus* didn't come off, I had decided there was one more attempt in me before I quit writing and did something else. I would spend 2006 writing one last novel, and if I didn't make it with that one, I was never going to. Looking back, I doubt I'd have written that next novel; it would have been World of Warcraft for God knows how long, back in the cocoon. The cocoon would perhaps have become too comfortable to emerge from at all.

Australian Literary Management were the first agency to get back in touch, early in the new year. This was big news. I forget exactly what was said, only that about halfway through, the call's significance hit me: *Lyn Tranter, one of the biggest, most established literary agents in the country, has called* you. *She's on the phone to* you, *right now.* I began stammering.

Lyn asked for the remainder of the manuscript. Recalling past disappointments, there was no cause yet to celebrate — only the risk of worse disappointment, like the drop from a greater height. When Lyn agreed to represent me, it was the biggest news I'd had yet. *Now* the inner pessimist shut his yap.

The twenty-eighth of February was the day of the announcement of the ABC Fiction Award winner. I had kept a casual eye on the approaching date, only because of the dream I'd had. When I got no phone call that day, it was disappointing, but at least I still had an agent, a very good one. I hadn't bothered to tell Lyn the manuscript was entered in the ABC competition — since the version I'd entered had been a tad less polished, there was no way I was winning … I'd never even pulled off a short-story competition win. I kept an eye on the competition only to see if I'd made the shortlist.

It turned out the response to the competition's first year had been overwhelming — nine hundred entries or so. Lots of old manuscripts dusted off, by the look of it.

That was a lot of reading for just four judges. They'd had to push the announcement date back.

Meanwhile, since I had an agent now, it was time to get serious again. I came out of my virtual vacation and began work on the next novel, *Nightfall*.

A phone call can change quite a bit in life, really. Jo Mackay, Commissioning Editor at ABC Books, rang on 15 March. Jo was also one of the judges of the competition, and the person who'd originally floated the idea of the award as a way to discover local authors.

I'd had a late night, a very late night, working on *Nightfall*, and although I knew that the ABC award's announcement had been pushed back, meaning I was technically still in the race, such a phone call was not what I'd expected to wake up to.

A woman on the other end of the line with an English accent introduced herself and said, 'Did you have an entry in the ABC Fiction Award?'

'Yes …' *Please don't hit me up for entry fees … I paid, surely I paid …*

'I've just called to tell you that you've won.'

Now then, this was a happy event, of course. Breaking the news to others was great, getting congratulatory emails and phone calls was great. Going to work after the announcement was like walking through a happy dream, handshakes from the boss and all that jazz.

That aside, when I had a little time to think about what came next, my reaction was one of terror. Long gone were any notions that I was a creature of any importance; hardly the subject of television, radio and newspaper articles.

But this award was to be publicised using all three. In two weeks, I'd be in Sydney talking to journalists from the major newspapers: the *Sydney Morning Herald*, the *Courier-Mail*, the *Australian* and others. There would be radio, including a live reading — Christ help me — and many interviews, even a brief television feature by the ABC's *Sunday Arts* program.

I had read somewhere that the publishing industry moves very slowly (and it does). On the assumption it would take time for my agent to find a publisher, more time yet for the book to actually be published, I'd expected maybe a year before any kind of limelight. But it was starting in *two weeks*.

In a panic I wrote to my agent and said I wanted to use a pseudonym. She asked why and I had a little trouble explaining. I paced through the apartment, terror feeding on itself, conjuring demons long buried.

STRANGE PLACES

It turned out there was less to worry about than I'd feared. Publicity comes in little bursts and then you're forgotten. Our best, most celebrated authors are probably surprised when they're recognised in the street, let alone newcomers like yours truly. (It has happened once, shortly after the book's launch; on a lunch break in the city, someone asked me if I was 'that book guy'.)

The launch was held at the Brisbane Writers' Festival that September. Jasper Fforde, the biggest name at the festival and an author I've admired for years, was a special guest, something I'll never forget. Something else I'll never forget is the look on my mother's face when she'd just bought the first copy ever to be bought, opened it, and saw the dedication.

At this time of writing, *Nightfall* hasn't yet been seriously submitted to publishers. That will be happening soon. *Nightfall* took the familiar formula to new extremes: this time, I began with conceptualizing the characters, *then* assembled a setting around them, the only kind of world (linked to ours) in which such an array of characters could possibly exist. That was a bold step — maybe too bold — but I am happy with the result. How the rest of the world feels about it will be revealed soon enough.

Nightfall was both a joy to work on, and my biggest test yet. It involved a struggle chiefly against myself as I succumbed to distractions and tried to put into perspective the fact that *Circus* found print, including idle months of abandoning the manuscript halfway through, convinced it was impossible to finish. At eighty thousand words, I declared *Nightfall* dead and buried, and began seeking other ideas, but could never quite shunt it out of my system. *If you can quit a novel at eighty thousand words, how can you know you'll ever finish the next one when the going gets hard?* was one question that got me working on it again, even after nearly six months away from it. Another factor was remembering I'd almost quit *Circus*, and it was only the fact that twenty thousand words were already invested that kept me going on it. Much of *Nightfall's* original content needed to be completely ripped out and rewritten, so that's what I did.

Now, I guess, it's time to start a new one.

I feel strange listing accolades — there are few ways to do it without sounding like a braggart or job applicant. But the ABC Fiction Award wasn't the end of the story for *The Pilo Family Circus*. Next there was the Aurealis Awards, luckily being held in Brisbane's Judith Wright Centre for Contemporary Arts. A few hundred industry people and fans of speculative fiction gathered on an absolutely sweltering February evening in 2007.

We all sat in a large lecture theatre. I'd hoped to win the Best Horror category, despite not having yet read my competitors' books. When it was announced I'd tied for the award with Edwina Grey's *Prismatic*, I was thrilled, but the tie certainly buried any hope of getting the Golden Aurealis. That was fine by me — I hadn't even considered *that* possibility. Andrew, who came along for the night tells me my reaction when they announced my book as the winner of the Golden Aurealis was an astonished expletive.

The Australian Shadows Award, presented by the Australian Horror Writers Association, was next. When the Ditmars — as the Australian Science Fiction Awards are known — rolled around, I had convinced myself it was impossible. If you're ever up for an award, I suggest this method — it seems to work. Later, thanks to the support of American spec fiction editor Ellen Datlow, I was shortlisted for the International Horror Guild Award. To see my name next to Stephen King's, among the other illustrious company on that list, was a feeling I struggle to articulate without puking up some kind of sappy cliché. So maybe I shouldn't try.

I was a touch bewildered by it all; I thought (and still think) that *Circus* is a book that does some things well, some things not so well. Maybe I've just had to read and rewrite the bloody thing once too often.

I've taken us almost up to the present moment. Right now we're having a rare cold snap in Queensland; it's like being on holiday. I've been more than eight months without a cigarette, thanks mostly to my lady friend, who expressed her distaste for the habit before we started dating. I feel a need to point this out to you because I've noticed in books that smoking characters often die before the book's end, and there's not much time remaining here …

Life as a published author has not resulted in delivery of a utopian key to a magical, better place, where life is without hassle. Hell, I'm still little better than broke. I expected otherwise, despite warnings, so if I feel denied or cheated, it's my own problem. Ultimately, not a whole lot has changed. I do love the job, but it's love-hate, and just lately, the last couple of years, I've hated it more than loved it. I don't know why — maybe because I've known nothing else for the last few years, nothing else at all. It's been an obsession, not a hobby, and that kind of wears you down. That will change, I expect. I can feel it changing already. The anticipation of my next project is pleasant; it doesn't carry with it the weight of dread and anxiety of recent times. It's not 'happily ever after' for me yet, but the night is young, and I think I'll get close enough, in the end.

And speaking of endings ... it is not with regret that I leave this manuscript be; I'd be telling fibs if I said this was the most fun I've ever had at the keyboard. You don't have to applaud or anything, but I'd like to thank you for reading.

AFTERWORD

So why me, huh? Damn you God, why did you bestow this curse upon me? Etcetera.

I felt that way, for a while. But there was something to consider. I've been to places that no one else on this planet will *ever* go, though of course others have had strange places to visit of their own. Me, I've lived for a short time as a werewolf. As a vampire. As a revolutionary. As a psychic. As a magician. As someone who cannot be hurt by physical force. As the uncoverer of conspiracies. As someone who can speak to the dead. As a rock star. As someone persecuted, hunted. I have lived in a police state. I have lived as Jesus Christ. I have been he who knows all. You see, all this is true. Because, for a while, it was all *real*.

Do you see what I mean?

What hurts, what really hurts, is that I will never feel so alive as I felt that night I ran barefoot from hospital, hearing vampires rustle in the trees above, hearing them swoop down to follow me, seeing a war zone around me, seeing battalions and guarded castles in the houses to either side of me, the air rife and thick with magic, some of it hostile, some of it benign, the air absolutely crackling with an energy that exists on the far boundary of the human mind, which, once crossed, we're not supposed to return from.

I made it back when I shouldn't have, so I'm lucky. But no matter what else happens in life, no matter what mountains I climb, no matter how close I come to death, whatever else I do, nothing will ever again make me feel so alive as I felt that night. Nothing.

THE PILO FAMILY CIRCUS

From the winner of five major literary awards, Will Elliott, comes *The Pilo Family Circus* ...

'You have two days to pass your audition. You better pass it feller, you're joining the circus. Ain't that the best news you ever got?'

Gonko on behalf of Doopy, Goshy, Winston and Rufshod. Clown division, Pilo Family Circus

The Pilo Family Circus is recruiting, and whether he likes it or not, share-house dweller and part-time concierge Jamie is auditioning.

He never wanted to join the circus but there's no refusing a troupe of malevolent headhunting clowns.

Before long, Jamie finds himself plunged into a nightmarish, centuries-old carnival, peopled by the gruesome, sadistic and savage a borderline world between earth and hell, full of comedic violence that is shadowed by a more sinister and ancient evil.

But worse is still to come. When Jamie daubs on his clown face-paint, he is transformed into the most vicious clown of all: JJ. And JJ wants Jamie dead.

'*The Pilo Family Circus* reminds us how far some Australian novelists have left the parochial behind.'
The Bulletin

Printed in Australia by Griffin Press
an Accredited ISO AS/NZS 14001:2004
Environmental Management System printer.